How to Stay Sane in Pain

CLARITY, RESILIENCE, AND CALM WITH LUPUS

KAREN DRENNAN-MCEWAN

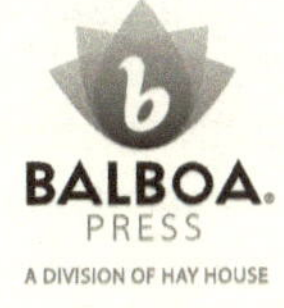

BALBOA.
PRESS
A DIVISION OF HAY HOUSE

Balboa Press books may be ordered through booksellers or by contacting:

Balboa Press
A Division of Hay House
1663 Liberty Drive
Bloomington, IN 47403
www.balboapress.com
1 (877) 407-4847

Print information available on the last page.

ISBN: 978-1-9822-2049-5 (sc)
ISBN: 978-1-9822-2051-8 (hc)
ISBN: 978-1-9822-2050-1 (e)

Library of Congress Control Number: 2019900743

Balboa Press rev. date: 02/15/2019

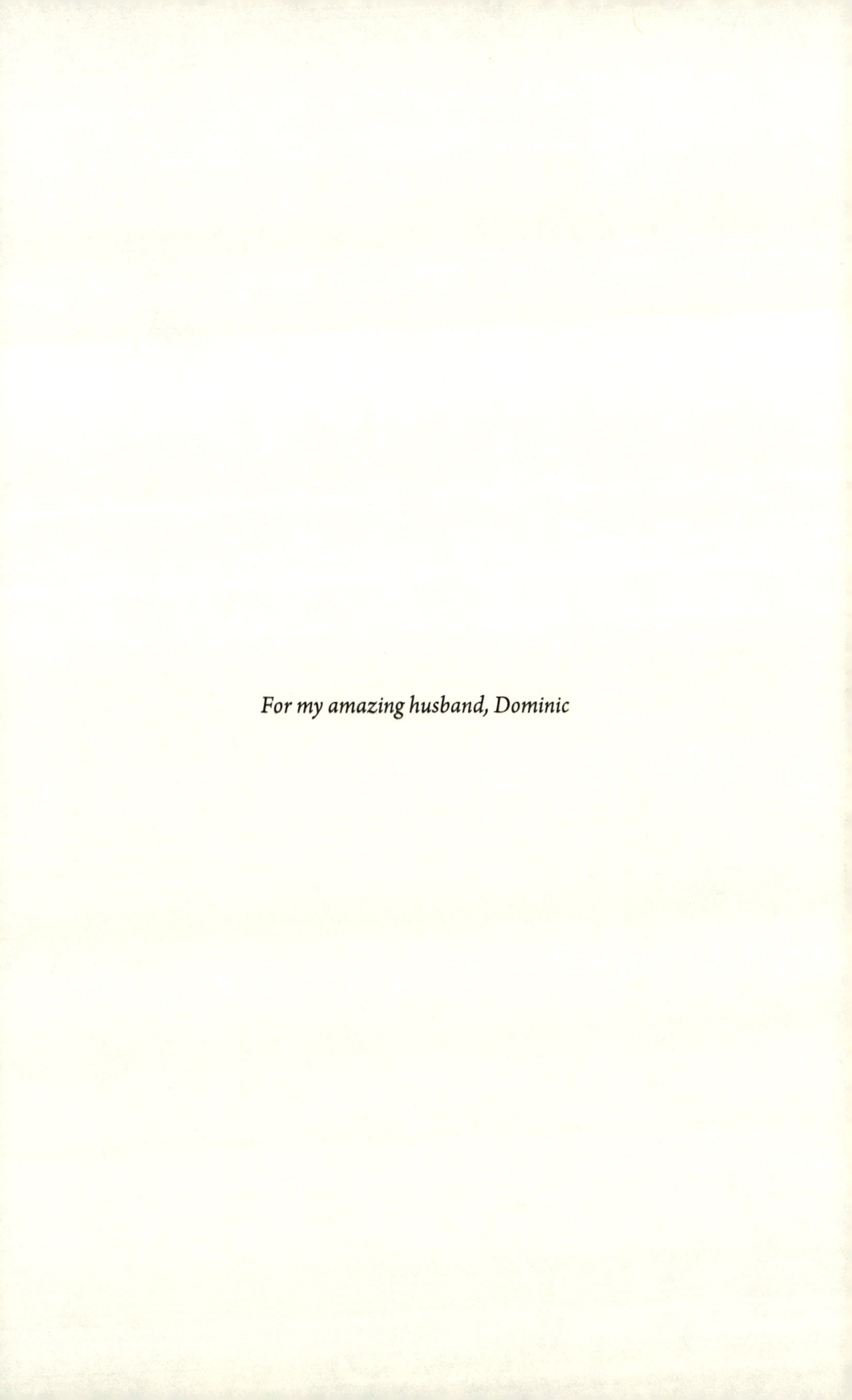

For my amazing husband, Dominic

CONTENTS

INTRODUCTION

> We read to know that we are not alone.
> —C. S. Lewis

This book was written by someone with lupus, with contributions from people with lupus, for people with lupus, and for those who love and care about them.

It is also for those who feel unwell right now but do not know what is wrong with them and are searching for the source of their mysterious symptoms. Similarly, you may be the loved one or friend of someone who seems to be suffering from a range of strange illnesses for which there appears to be no answer.

Some 1.5 million Americans have been diagnosed with lupus, and it is estimated that approximately 5 million people worldwide currently have the disease. The majority with lupus have systemic lupus erythematosus (SLE), which impacts the whole body, while some 10 percent have discoid lupus erythematosus (DLE), which primarily involves the skin.

Systemic lupus erythematosus, in particular, is not neatly diagnosed. No one or two clear symptoms are decisive, and lupus is often described as "mimicking" other diseases. It has mild, moderate, and severe forms; and the path of the condition can vary from remission and dormancy to periods of heightened disease activity, known as "flares." Systemic lupus erythematosus does in fact have a small group of telltale symptoms, but at present, the disease is unfamiliar to most and widely misunderstood. This lack of understanding is leading to high levels of misdiagnosis, belated diagnosis, and downright wrong diagnosis of the disease. Therefore, this could be one of the leading "sleeper" diseases of modern times, with people suffering from systemic lupus erythematosus, unacknowledged and untreated.

Why is this important? Well, because unrecognized and unmedicated, it can progress stealthily to threaten major organs—and thereby people's lives and also the lives of unborn children. Lupus pregnancies are now routinely designated "high risk," and the majority of those who are diagnosed are women of childbearing age.

Although mild lupus can be well controlled by medication, moderate and severe lupus can be debilitating and life-changing, as this book will show. Patients often struggle against a lack of knowledge about the severity of symptoms and the progress of the disease. There have been great advances in the modern medical management of the disease in the last seventy years, but a permanent cure has yet to be found.

While efforts to raise awareness of the condition continue to increase, there is clearly much more to be done. Some celebrity cases in recent years—including Seal, Selena Gomez, and Lady Gaga—have raised the profile, but more education and publicity is certainly needed.

I was admitted to the hospital for treatment for a severe infection in 2012, unaware that many of the illnesses experienced throughout my life had in fact been lupus symptoms and that in preceding months, the disease had been progressing, quietly wreaking damage to my internal organs.

What I also did not know that first night in the hospital was that the infection had just ignited a dangerous lupus flare that would rage through my body, leaving me emaciated, life-threateningly weak, in a wheelchair, and in constant pain within weeks.

Once diagnosed with severe systemic lupus erythematosus, it became clear that I had a medical condition with a strange name that was not widely understood. Indeed, it was to become apparent that it was a complex disease and answers were scattered and often not easily available. This book aims to address those multiple queries, which, from examining the forums on the Internet and interviewing fellow lupus patients, are shared worldwide.

This multifaceted condition needs a multifaceted approach. Incorporating the stories of others with lupus and referring to the latest research, this narrative is divided into three easy parts, namely medical, psychological, and complementary physical. Part I, "Understanding Lupus," gives a comprehensive understanding of lupus, from how it is diagnosed, through its medical history, to its leading symptoms and medications and their main side effects.

Part II, "A Mental and Emotional Journey," recognizes the psychological implications of living with lupus. Given my training and experience as a counsellor and psychotherapist, I was in a better position than many. Nevertheless, I still had to ride the lupus mental roller coaster. Recognition and validation of these tumultuous feelings would have helped at the time, and clarification would have bolstered my shattered confidence. This book aims to give you that reassurance by detailing the psychological toll of medications and the disease, with contributions from others with lupus to complete the picture.

Part II then goes on to give you the psychotherapeutic solutions that I used to survive, to recover my equilibrium and gain a new sense of purpose and joy in life, despite chronic pain and debilitating symptoms. It shows exactly how to employ tried-and-tested cognitive behavioral techniques including positive reframing, rebuilding and rescheduling, together with mindfulness, guided meditations, and visualizations. It is a systematic guide to changing your mind-set, renewing your sense of achievement and purpose, and creating mental calm, despite hugely challenging circumstances. This part in particular may also be helpful to those suffering from pain and chronic illness due to causes other than lupus.

A holistic approach is, according to the dictionary, characterized by "the belief that parts of something are intimately connected and explicable only by reference to the whole." The physical and mental benefits of parts I and II are consolidated in part III, "Holistic Physical Solutions," which firstly is a guide to sensible and achievable nutrition for lupus and shows what to avoid and what to add to your diet. Secondly, Part III describes those complementary physical therapies that reinforce the psychological work carried out and add benefits and healing not covered by mainstream medical treatment.

These three parts come together to form a holistic methodology that combines the best of modern medicine with psychotherapeutic techniques, optimum dietary advice, and the most suitable complementary treatments. The result is a powerful mind-body approach specifically tailored to this difficult disease.

If what I learned can benefit even a few other people who are going through what I have experienced, or worse, or can help the loved ones or friends of those in pain and suffering, then my aims will have been achieved.

Ultimately, I have set out to give the information and guidance that I really needed when my lupus flared out of control. I am evidence that this approach is both necessary and beneficial, and this is the story of my journey.

PART I

Understanding Lupus

CHAPTER 1

A Sudden Reversal

Life is what happens to you while you are busy making other plans.
—"Beautiful Boy," John Lennon

Jolted awake, I found myself propped up against starched white pillows in a London hospital bed. A partially open door percolated determined footsteps and the rattle of trollies from the corridor outside. Diffused early-morning light filtered through a square window facing out onto a giant internal well. I could see nothing green, just floor upon floor of gray concrete walls and opaque glass, with spring rain falling down from the sky.

On emergency admission the previous afternoon, my temperature had been high, 103.6 degrees Fahrenheit, and my stomach was so swollen with fluid that it made me look six months pregnant. With kind and reassuring nurses checking my vital signs hourly throughout the night, sleep was fleeting. In addition, the open door was evidence of their concern. Feeling strangely stiff and heavily restricted by intravenous needles attached to tubes connected to pouches of fluid, and with clips delivering oxygen into my nose, I reached out for the call button resting on the edge of the table next to the bed. It was a little orange circle with the outline of a nurse on it. Normally, pressing it would have been a simple task. However, I found that rotating my right elbow and moving my arm proved so startlingly painful that I could only inch across the bedsheet toward my goal.

Finally reaching the button, my forefinger had hardly any strength left to press down, and it hit home that a system designed for sick people was almost beyond me. The source of the intense pain and pathetic weakness was unknown. I had not been like this yesterday. The nurses tutted and frowned slightly. They rapidly added another pouch of clear fluid to the pole, and pain relief began to drip steadily down into my arm.

On day two, a livid red rash spread across my lower cheeks on either side of my nose, so deep on the left side that it dragged the skin downward. Smaller roundish red patches decorated the base of my neck and across my collarbones like an unwelcome necklace.

Tests began and continued daily, with blood tests with and an MRI, up and down through the hospital in lifts to different floors in a wheelchair, knees covered in a rug. The blood tests showed serious damage to my liver. This was not a surprise, for it had been under investigation by the liver consultant who admitted me. However, the MRI also discovered that my spleen had vanished. Unsure what that meant exactly, I simply parked any sense of unease in the mental check-back-later file.

My stiff hands were cramped inward, rigid and bent, particularly my dominant right hand. Down in physiotherapy, they pried open the stiffened fingers and placed them around a softball, which they made me squeeze repeatedly. I returned exhausted from the sessions. And despite the therapists' efforts, I continued to find holding cutlery extremely challenging; cutting with a knife was virtually impossible. Too embarrassed to ask for help, I struggled with my meals.

On day five, my liver consultant took off his smart raincoat and perched on the end of my bed. "Well, given all your symptoms and the negative results for ..." He reeled off a list of truly frightening-sounding diseases. "I personally would start to treat you for something called lupus." I nodded, vaguely recognizing the word but in total ignorance of much else.

"I said that your liver problems were a symptom, not the cause. And given what we have learned, I believe the cause is most likely lupus." He paused and took a deep breath. "Now, I could start treating you for this, but given that we have a specialist lupus team linked to this hospital, it seems ridiculous for me, a liver specialist, to treat you when they are here. So I am going to try to get you an appointment with them as soon as possible, although they are super busy because they are one of the best centers in the world for lupus."

Despite my request, he was reluctant to allow me to go home, but I negotiated a review in twenty-four hours instead. He left in a swirl of tan gabardine, and the rain continued to slide down the window.

A day later, in preparation for my departure, a nurse came, detached the painkiller drip, and presented me with a single white tablet in a little paper cup. "You need to get used to being on a lower level of pain medication for when you go home," she said with an emphatic nod.

I eyed the large lone tablet with suspicion, instinctively doubtful. This was to prove a lesson in listening to my intuition. Three hours later, the pain in my limbs was so bad that it made me feel nauseated, and this escalated until a compassionate nurse injected me with an antiemetic. The pouch of pain relief was then quickly returned to my intravenous infusion pole and reconnected without comment.

Mentally and emotionally, it was a strange bubble. Outwardly, I waited patiently and calmly, but internally I felt they were all rather overreacting. Looking back, I appreciate the denial about the seriousness of my situation and acknowledge my dismissiveness as a coping mechanism.

Finally allowed to go home, tucked into the car, surrounded by pillows to protect me from bumps in the road, and dosed up with strong muscle relaxants, I pointed to the red marks on my cheek. "It isn't that bad," my husband said; however, from his sideways look, I knew instantly that it was very bad indeed.

Reaching the house, I was eased out of the car and supported into the hall. In greeting, the terrier panted and bounced around in circles, while the young bird dog left the ground entirely in her excitement.

Despite my bravado, my daily routine saw me shuffling, weak as a kitten, between the bed and the sofa to watch television or sleeping propped up for hours on end. A half-seated position with my shoulders supported and my legs raised proved the most comfortable, with a rug for warmth and a dog curled up at the end of the sofa to keep me company. I was unable to do much for myself; I did not even have the strength to lift a kettle to make a cup of tea, let alone prepare food or cook. I needed someone permanently on hand to take care of me and to pick up all the tasks that I had previously completed without a second's thought. It became increasingly clear this was no nasty bug or even the flu—tough for a few days, a fortnight even, and then recovery sets in. I waited in vain to wake up feeling suddenly clearer and stronger. Denial did not appear to be working.

Little did I know this would turn out to be only the beginning of a long road for me and those close to me. The life I was previously living had come to an immediate and devastating halt.

CHAPTER 2

The Route to Diagnosis

To strive, to seek, to find and not to yield.
—Alfred, Lord Tennyson

Remarkably, my liver consultant got me an appointment with the specialist lupus unit on the Monday after my departure from the hospital the previous Friday. My new London lupus consultant told me he would not treat me for lupus without further blood and muscle tests. Despite the fact that I was in a wheelchair, he said he could offer no new medicine or additional help until these were completed. Facing the prospect of more days in this weak condition and experiencing such pain frightened me. I sensed myself slipping further and further downward, and I broke down into rare tears in front of him. Nevertheless, he remained adamant that without further tests, his hands were tied.

An electromyography (EMG) is performed to assess weakness in the muscles and identify neuromuscular abnormalities, aiming to detect true weakness as opposed to that resulting from pain or reduced motivation (Leis and Schenk 2018). It can be done on an inpatient or outpatient basis. This involved a separate trip four days later, again bundled to and from the country to London in the car. When the doctor opened his door to see me waiting outside in my wheelchair with my husband, he looked shocked and perplexed. "There must be some mistake. I am treating outpatients, not inpatients, today."

I clearly looked so unwell that he immediately assumed I must be hospitalized and was not capable of journeying in from home. Climbing onto his couch for testing proved excruciating and took the better part of five minutes. He concluded, perhaps not surprisingly, that my muscles were indeed seriously impaired.

Diagnosing lupus is complex. The overall picture is confused by the fact there are mild, moderate, and severe forms. Across many platforms, it is frequently described as "masquerading" as other diseases. Officially, there are four types of lupus. Systemic lupus erythematosus, or SLE, is the most common, at around 80 percent of cases; cutaneous or discoid lupus erythematosus, or DLE, which primarily impacts the skin, accounts for about 10 percent of cases. There are also two much rarer kinds, namely drug-induced lupus, where symptoms usually subside when the drugs are stopped; and the even rarer neonatal lupus, where the mother's antibodies trigger rashes, liver difficulties, or low blood cell counts in the infant. Symptoms typically go away after about six months, with no long-term effects.

This book focuses on systemic lupus erythematosus, but it also discusses discoid lupus where helpful. Throughout the book, the generic term *lupus* is used, and there is a natural emphasis on SLE because it is the most common and has the most varied symptoms.

Medical personnel thrust pamphlets into your hands as you leave appointments, and lupus centers around the world often have comprehensive information on their websites. No one source has all the answers, nor do some doctors in the limited confines of a consultation. The result is that you can end up feeling bombarded by tests with inadequate explanations, creating a deep sense of bewilderment.

The reality is that it took me years to understand why it took so long for my doctors to reach a conclusion, why there were so many different tests, and for me to learn what constitutes an official diagnosis for lupus. There is no doubt in my mind that this lack of clarity only adds to the lupus patient's sense of uncertainty. If you combine strange symptoms, mix in inexplicable fatigue, add a great deal of pain, and then top it all up with a high dose of mystery, then it is not surprising that many in the process of being diagnosed feel completely overwhelmed.

An Official Diagnosis

Undoubtedly, it would have helped me to understand the process by which lupus is medically diagnosed. I eventually stumbled across the modern checklist against which symptoms have to be assessed by doctors to give an official diagnosis of systemic lupus erythematosus or discoid lupus erythematosus with systemic complications. It turns out that one lupus symptom on its own is not conclusive and that a certain number of boxes need to be ticked to add up to a positive result. On this official list are eleven symptoms that are indicative of systemic lupus erythematosus, and at least four of these criteria must be met.

Below are the key criteria for an official diagnosis so you don't have to wonder as I did. You will still have to suffer the tests and await the results, but understanding this step at the outset would have clarified matters for me enormously. In this situation, ignorance is *not* bliss.

The following are the American College of Rheumatology (ACR) diagnostic criteria, which are remembered in the mnemonic "SOAP BRAIN MD":

- **S**erositis, or inflammation, of key tissues such as those lining the lungs, heart, and abdomen
- **O**ral ulcers
- **A**rthritis, as in tenderness and swelling of the joints
- **P**hotosensitivity
- **B**lood disorders
- **R**enal (kidney) involvement
- **A**ntinuclear antibodies
- **I**mmunologic phenomena—for example, anti-dsDNA antibodies
- **N**eurologic disorders of the nerves, brain, and spine
- **M**alar rash
- **D**iscoid rash

(Bartels 2017)

<u>Serositis</u>

This is where the thin layers of serous or serosal fluid, which allows major organs such as the lungs, the abdomen, and the heart to move smoothly within the body, become inflamed. Research estimates that some 50 percent of systemic lupus erythematosus patients will experience some form of lung involvement during the course of their condition. According to the Johns Hopkins Lupus Center, the five main problems are "pleuritic, acute lupus pneumonitis, chronic (fibrotic) lupus pneumonitis, pulmonary arterial hypertension, and shrinking lung syndrome." The lungs are involved when there is pain when deep breathing, laughing, coughing, or sneezing, which can be when the visceral pleura, or lining, is inflamed. Acute cases of lupus pneumonitis can instigate a dry cough, bringing up blood.

It is essential to report any unusual lung pains or symptoms to your doctor in order to be treated with corticosteroids/and or immunosuppressants early to prevent permanent scarring of the lungs. Lupus can also inflame the lining of the abdomen and the organs within, leading to tenderness, swelling, fluid retention, and aches and pains. Heart involvement can involve all components of the heart, and symptoms can include chest discomfort, ranging from the mild to the severe. An electrocardiogram may be required (Moder 1999).

Oral Ulcers

Ulcers in the mouth and on the tongue and sores in the nose are primary symptoms of lupus but are usually painless. They can present in multiples of four to six and upward at any one time. "Oral lesions (oral ulcers, ulcerative plaques) in the context of lupus erythematosus have long been described" (Nico 2008).

Arthritis—Swollen and Tender Joints

Throughout the body, joints can become painfully inflamed, red, and swollen, feeling tender and stiff and either warm or cold to the touch. Those farthest from the body are often the most targeted: fingers and toes, wrists, ankles, knees, and elbows. Pain in the hips and shoulders can also be present. Ultimately, and this point truly needs to be stressed, the combination of rashes with swollen or painful joints is a particular marker for lupus.

<u>Photosensitivity</u>

"Two thirds of people with lupus have increased sensitivity to ultraviolet rays, either from sunlight or from artificial inside light—or both" (Werth 2017). Discoid rashes are sensitive to sunlight, often appearing on exposed areas such as the face, hands, and neck. This is why patients are advised on diagnosis of both systemic lupus erythematosus and discoid lupus to stay out of the sun, to cover up with clothing and hats, and to wear high-factor sunscreen. The sunscreen needs to be broad spectrum, providing both UVA and UVB coverage, and at least factor 15 or more for general wear and factor 30 or more for extended outdoor activity. Otherwise, in addition to skin rashes, patients may experience itching and burning sensations. The exposure to the sun can also manifest flares in underlying systemic symptoms such as joint pain and fatigue (Bowman and Spriggs 2016).

<u>Ian's Story</u>

Ian wrote to me about his problems with sun exposure in the years before his eventual diagnosis with lupus: "For years, I was sure the doctor thought I was a bit soft, always saying my hands are sore, this is sore, that is sore. When I went out, I was told that I was boring or antisocial due to being knackered. Holidays were not looked forward to, as I was just waiting for some sort of infection to start due to the sun, which I had no idea was making me worse!" Being a carpenter and working outside often, Ian has had to continue to be very careful about his sun protection.

The wrong kind of internal lighting can trigger or worsen skin rashes and can set off other systemic symptoms such as joint pain, weakness, fatigue, headaches, or migraines. While working in London in my early thirties, I moved to a new job as a stockbroker, with one of the attractions of the role being that my team's section of the dealing room overlooked the Thames River and was therefore flooded with natural light. However, some eight months after moving to the new job, one of the original family owners of the firm, a director, fancied the view instead and forced thirteen different departments to move around in order for him to acquire it.

My department then found itself in a dark corner, and I spent long city hours working under old-style overhead UV strip lighting. I started to get severe migraines. In retrospect, it is probable that these were a result of my underlying lupus. Luckily, moving to a new job some months later and subsequently always working in offices lit by natural light, the migraines did not return, even though it was to be over fifteen years before my lupus was officially diagnosed.

Blood Disorders

The presence of anti-double stranded DNA (anti-dsDNA) in the blood is a clear marker because it is hardly ever present in people who do not have lupus. This is why it is one of the tests needing to be positive to confirm an official diagnosis. Interestingly, this test shows an increased level of the marker when the lupus is more active, so it can also be used as a means of monitoring the progression of the condition.

The erythrocyte sedimentation rate (ESR) test is a blood test measuring the level of inflammation in the body, and inflammation is often raised in lupus sufferers. Therefore, again, it is often used to monitor the condition.

Lupus can often influence the number of white and red blood cells present in a patient's blood. A low amount of hemoglobin present can indicate anemia, with the platelet count showing whether the disease or any of the drugs being taken are adversely targeting the bone marrow.

The inherent variability of lupus can also complicate the process of blood testing, in that some tests may come up inconclusive and then read positive a week or so later. Hence, in some cases, repeated tests may be necessary for a conclusive diagnosis. Once diagnosed, regular monitoring is a given.

Renal Disorders

If not controlled and allowed to go unchecked, systemic lupus erythematosus can damage the major organs of the body. Doctors can use liver function tests, urine tests, kidney filtration tests, X-rays, ultrasounds, and CT (computed tomography) or MRI (magnetic resonance imaging) scans to check, in combination with blood analysis and also sometimes with biopsies.

Selena Gomez, the international pop star, has received publicity for her lupus, which made her gravely ill in 2017 after attacking her kidneys. This led to her undergoing a kidney transplant donated by her friend Francia Raisa Almendarez later in that year.

Antinuclear Antibodies

People diagnosed with lupus, as noted in the official list, can have various distinctive blood disorders, and of particular note is the presence of antinuclear antibodies (ANAs). Some 98 percent of people with lupus have these antibodies, but so do people without, so their presence does not confirm lupus on their own. However, they do become part of the diagnostic jigsaw puzzle that produces a positive diagnosis.

Immunologic Phenomenon

This describes the presence of a range of antibodies in a lupus patient's blood, with the two most commonly discussed antibodies being the lupus anticoagulant (LA) and the anticardiolipin antibody (aCL), both of which are antiphospholipid antibodies. Over 50 percent of lupus patients have antiphospholipid antibodies in their blood. There is further detail on antiphospholipid antibodies in the section on the history of lupus.

Peculiarities in blood tests can also extend to lupus patients being incorrectly diagnosed with other diseases, especially if other signs of lupus are not recognized or symptoms are not presenting at the time because of a lull in lupus activity. The most notable of these false positives is highlighted by research that has shown that some 20 percent of lupus patients will present with a false-positive test for syphilis. In other words, while they have these antibodies present, they are a sign of lupus rather than syphilis.

I came across just such an example when I met a lupus patient who had been incorrectly diagnosed with syphilis by a random test while accompanying a friend to a London sexually transmitted disease (STD) clinic. Remarkably, despite having no other symptoms at the time, she received full treatment for syphilis. In addition, she had to contact previous partners, who in turn had to be tested. Some months later, going to another doctor with severe limb pain, a facial rash, and acute tiredness, she happened to mention the positive syphilis test as part of the consultation. This doctor, aware of the lupus blood markers, instantly made the correct link. Then, with the suite of other lupus blood tests completed, a diagnosis of systemic lupus erythematosus could finally be confirmed and treatment for the correct condition begun. Research from 2012 concluded the following: "Chronic false-positive Venereal Disease Research Laboratory (VDRL) test results are relatively common in patients with autoimmune disorders" (Hook 2012).

Much rarer examples of false positives of the human immunodeficiency virus type 1 (HIV1) have also been recorded (Jindal 1993).

Neurologic Disorders

Lupus can cause problems in the central nervous system and with peripheral nerves. According to research, central nervous reactions can include balance issues, headaches, vision problems, seizures, and even strokes. Peripheral neuropathy damage can lead to tingling, numbness, and shooting pain in the extremities, particularly to the hands and feet. Referral to a neurologist for lupus patients is common.

Malar Rash

The malar, or butterfly, rash—pale pink or bright red in color—spreads over the nose and then across both cheeks. It is perhaps the leading distinctive mark of lupus but is not present in all cases. It can be worse on one cheek than on the other and therefore not a symmetrical butterfly shape with open wings, and it can be raised or flat. There is research to suggest that it can be one of the first signs of the onset of a lupus flare, although transient and fading not long after but leaving other systemic symptoms in place. My malar rash, classic in shape but worse on the left, where it included a deep lesion, also disappeared within about six weeks after initial hospitalization. It left an indented scar on my left cheek where the lesion had been. I have also interviewed lupus patients who live with almost permanent light red rashes over their noses and cheeks.

A high-profile celebrity example of lupus is pop star Seal Samuel, better known simply as Seal, who has distinctive deep scars on his cheeks. For many years, I thought his scars were some sort of cool statement, but after my diagnosis and reading widely, I discovered that he had in fact suffered from discoid lupus erythematosus as a teenager, and although his lupus has been in remission for many years, the deep scars remain.

<u>Discoid Rash</u>

Discoid rashes are red, roughly circular, and usually have a slightly raised rim. In milder cases, they can look like pale leopard spots. Confusingly, they are present in both discoid and systemic lupus, but as previously identified, discoid lupus erythematosus normally only affects the skin, usually from the neck and above, and does not target anywhere else in the body. It is estimated that discoid lupus erythematosus only becomes systemic lupus erythematosus in about 10 percent of cases, but this is caveated by acknowledgment that the patient may have had the systemic form all along, with the rash being the first recognizable symptom. A point clarified by research concluded the following: "Discoid lupus patients who have not developed clinically significant SLE manifestations within the first two years of the appearance of their skin lesions have a very low risk of suffering from severe systemic lupus erythematosus (SLE) complications later in their disease course" (Sontheimer 1989).

As mentioned, my discoid rashes appeared down my neck and across my collarbone and were at their worst, red and raised, upon leaving the hospital for the first time. They have flared back up to a lesser degree numerous times since, often accompanied by heightened fatigue, before fading again. They can leave pale patches on the skin by way of scars, but mine proved more superficial than the malar rash.

As we progress, I will describe other symptoms typical of lupus that can also arise when you have the condition, but for now, this is the list of key markers needed for an official diagnosis.

Overlapping Autoimmune Conditions

Lupus is also part of a group of autoimmune diseases that can coexist to a greater or lesser extent with the condition. These so-called comorbidities can add further complexity. Michael Lockshin concluded in 2015, "Overlapping autoimmune disease is common in patients with SLE." The leading autoimmune disorders that can often coexist with lupus include, in alphabetical order, the following:

- Chronic fatigue syndrome: This is also known as myalgic encephalomyelitis, or ME.
- Diabetes: In type 1 diabetes, the immune system attacks the insulin-producing beta cells in the pancreas and destroys them.
- Fibromyalgia.
- Graves' disease: This is often the underlying cause of hypothyroidism, where the thyroid gland at the front of the neck produces too much thyroid hormone. It is typified by a swollen neck, previously known as goiter, and sometimes protuberant eyes as well.
- Hashimoto's disease: This is the reverse of Graves' disease in that the thyroid gland is damaged and causes weight gain, tiredness, and depression.
- Inflammatory bowel diseases such as Crohn's disease and celiac disease.
- Multiple sclerosis.
- Psoriasis.
- Raynaud's syndrome.
- Rheumatoid arthritis (RA).
- Sjögren's syndrome.

The leading comorbidities are fibromyalgia, Raynaud's syndrome, rheumatoid arthritis, and Sjögren's syndrome.

<u>Fibromyalgia</u>

It is estimated that some 30 percent of lupus patients also suffer from fibromyalgia. This condition is not fully understood. It leads to widespread and often intense pain at eighteen possible points across the body, with sensitivity and pain occurring at the same time on either side of the body in nine matching areas of "the neck, shoulders, chest, hips, knees, and elbows," according to the Lupus Foundation of America.

Raynaud's Syndrome

Raynaud's syndrome is also estimated to impact about 30 percent of people with lupus. In cold conditions, the body's normal response is to prioritize keeping the body's core and major organs warm, but with Raynaud's this process overreacts. As a result, the extremities (fingers and toes) suffer, but sometimes the ears, nose, lips, and chin do as well. These can become extremely pale, often turning white or blue in color, and can feel numb or prickly. Then, as the body warms up again, the blood flows back, also in excess, causing redness, swelling, and sometimes sharp pain.

Rheumatoid Arthritis

Approximately another 30 percent of SLE patients will also have rheumatoid arthritis, the combination of which is sometimes referred to as "rhupus." Although both are autoimmune conditions, there are key differences between the two. Firstly, rheumatoid arthritis is focused on the joints, especially the hands, whereas lupus can influence many aspects of the body as well as cause painful and swollen joints. Secondly, rheumatoid arthritis manifests in both sides of the body symmetrically, like fibromyalgia, while lupus can target one side of the body or one particular joint and not others. Finally, rheumatoid arthritis leads to erosion of the joints, while, despite the pain, lupus does not progressively damage the joints.

Sjögren's Syndrome

Sjögren's syndrome is named after Henrik Sjögren (1899–1976), a Swedish ophthalmologist. It adversely targets the fluid-producing functions of the body: tears and saliva. Its main symptoms are dry eyes and a dry mouth, but it can also cause joint and muscle pain and fatigue. Secondary symptoms can include swollen glands, rashes, and numbness or weakness in the hands and feet. A high-profile case of Sjögren's is tennis champion Venus Williams, who was diagnosed in 2011. Again, Sjögren's often coexists with other autoimmune conditions and appears in about 30 percent of lupus cases.

The syndrome is treated most commonly with eye lubricant drops and saliva-promoting tablets or prednisolone or immunosuppressants if these prove insufficient. The symptoms of dry eyes, namely soreness, burning, grittiness, and irritation can be helped with a range of preservative free drops following an ophthalmological test or a dry-eye consultation with an optometrist. Eye drops containing *Hamamelis virginiana* (common or American witch hazel) can also be obtained over the counter. Massaging around the eye socket using your forefingers in small circular movements can also prove helpful.

Your doctor can also prescribe saliva-supporting tablets for the relief of dry mouth symptoms. On return from the hospital, I began to suffer from a dry mouth, but my lips were also so dry and cracked that they bled. Mouth problems are indicative of systemic lupus erythematosus, so this is something of a crossover symptom.

You can see from the math that it is not uncommon for lupus patients to have one or more overlapping syndromes. For some, the presence of these other diseases can make diagnosis even more complex.

Lupus can also move between periods when symptoms are low and more under control to periods when activity is more intense. It is also clear that the disease can retreat into periods of dormancy, sometimes for years, before becoming active again. These active phases are called lupus "flares." The firefighting analogy gives you the sense that, like a fire, lupus can smolder away before something apparently unrelated, like a puff of wind, can whip it up into an inferno. Viral or bacterial infections or even simple stress have been identified as the culprits for igniting the underlying condition into flares.

Unfortunately, all these variables, combined with lack of familiarity with the distinctive symptoms, are leading to widespread non-diagnosis, misdiagnosis, belated diagnosis, and downright wrong diagnosis of this condition. The majority of the fellow systemic lupus erythematosus patients whom I have spoken to and corresponded with have spent years frustrated and misunderstood. In their search for an accurate diagnosis, some have even been advised by their doctors to seek counselling/psychological support or have been prescribed antidepressants.

I have come across stories where a patient was on antidepressants for seven years prior to a successful diagnosis of lupus, and also of a patient, with a successful career in the armed forces behind her, who was offered counselling after repeated visits to her general practitioner failed to identify the true cause of her symptoms. It is evident that because of non-diagnosis, psychosomatic causes are at times being blamed instead. Even worse, some with unrecognized lupus cases are being judged as hypochondriacs. The woman with the armed forces background eventually collapsed with such severe pain and swelling that she was rushed to accident and emergency with suspected meningitis before being finally diagnosed with severe systemic lupus erythematosus.

Obviously, as a trained psychotherapist, I am now wholly supportive of having counselling and psychological assistance for the mental and emotional challenges that lupus presents, in addition to antidepressants if necessary where there has been a correctly assessed clinical need. Furthermore, I advocate psychological solutions for dealing with the mental implications of lupus in the second part of this book. Nevertheless, psychotherapy cannot, and definitely should not, replace an accurate diagnosis and the correct medical analysis and treatment that this brings.

A medical diagnosis and ongoing monitoring must be the foundation upon which all other interventions are built. Long-term non-diagnosis perpetuates uncontrolled disease activity, which can harm the major organs and be life-threatening, as "early damage can increase mortality risk" (Pego-Reigosa 2016). The whole premise of this book is that psychological solutions and complementary physical therapies, which are described in parts II and III, should work in conjunction with first-rate conventional medical treatment. Therefore, a correct medical diagnosis is an essential starting point.

Failure to recognize the symptoms of lupus and to diagnose it correctly is currently nothing short of endemic, and I do not use that word lightly. Recent research by the Lupus Foundation of America in 2017 showed that out of a study of 3,022 adults with lupus in the United States, 41.0 percent reported being misdiagnosed with something other than lupus at the start of their journey. This study discovered that nearly 40 percent of the participants had waited over a year for an accurate diagnosis. This is despite the fact that some 34.5 percent of the respondents were reported as having "severe symptoms," while, amazingly, 13.3 percent had symptoms that were "life-threatening."

In the study, 93.5 percent of the respondents were female, 6.5 percent were male, and 86.2 percent were adults between the ages of twenty-five and sixty-four years. Astonishingly, over half of the sample, 54.1 percent, had been told initially that there was nothing wrong with them or that their symptoms were psychological.

Unsurprisingly, the authors concluded that their report identified the need for "ongoing education" about lupus. Paola Daly, director of research at the Lupus Foundation of America, said, "This study is so valuable because it is the first in-depth look at the patient diagnostic experience and the results of this survey will help us to understand and, in turn, prevent the specific factors that lead to unacceptable delays in receiving a lupus diagnosis."

A separate study by Lupus UK from a survey of its membership, with 2,527 responses, reported in 2018, "It is taking on average 6.4 years to diagnose lupus from the first symptoms experienced." This lack of awareness, although perhaps entirely understandable, is potentially dangerous. Given the evidence of widespread ignorance of some of the characteristics of the disease within the medical community itself, let alone within the wider population, there is every possibility that there are people who are unaware that they have lupus. This is why systemic lupus could yet prove to be a leading hidden illness of the modern era.

A telephone call from a medical secretary in London confirmed that my tests had come back positive for a diagnosis of systemic lupus erythematosus. She also confirmed the diagnosis as severe, rather than moderate or mild.

It was explained that this was a lifelong condition for which there was currently no cure. Nonetheless, armed with a diagnosis, my medical history finally became clearer. I pieced together many anomalies, tracking back and identifying periods when the lupus had been more active as well as when it must have gone dormant before flaring again. More recently, it had clearly been ticking along undiscovered, giving me aches and stiffness in the mornings and silently attacking internal organs. This time it had destroyed my spleen, the official term being *auto infarct*, and had been seriously damaging my liver before the infection had supercharged it into a massive flare.

Ultimately, with the diagnosis of systemic lupus erythematosus confirmed, my initial feelings were of overwhelming relief. Finally being able to put a name to my ill health felt, in itself, a watershed moment.

My research has come across numerous examples of patients making multiple visits, often to several different doctors, only to be told that there is nothing wrong with them. Interviews and correspondence with these people has verified that their eventual diagnosis has given them welcome clarity. Confirmation has proved mentally and emotionally beneficial: no longer disbelieved, they feel vindicated, and whatever they face, they feel far better to be aware of it than in the dark.

Knowing that targeted treatment could now begin, I had confidence that with the right medicine, these terrible symptoms would subside. I regretted the loss of my spleen, which made me now more susceptible to infections, but took the optimistic view that it could have been much worse. I had previously been incorrectly diagnosed with bone marrow cancer after a peculiar set of blood tests. Years of strange symptoms and unexplained illnesses were now solved, and knowing my enemy felt more empowering than facing an unseen opponent.

CHAPTER 3

Discovering Lupus

The past is the present unrolled for understanding.
—Will Durant, *The Lessons of History*

So with spring well under way, I found myself finally successfully diagnosed with a condition that had a very strange name and which the majority of people had never heard of. More particularly, I knew almost nothing about it either!

These were among some of the first questions I had: Who else has it? How rare is it? What causes it? I did not know answers to any of these questions at the outset. From current evidence on the lupus forums, this continues to be the case for many recently diagnosed patients. Initially so ill, I could only speculate for months, but eventually I began to collect answers from a huge variety of e-books and online sources (the most helpful of which are listed at the back of this book). It would have been better not to have to try to gather information here and there while in the grip of a life-changing condition. Instead, it would have been much more reassuring to have the main points answered in layman's language in one place. For your clarity and reassurance, it is my intention to give you the comfort of knowing what you are dealing with and share the pointers that I lacked.

It is estimated that approximately 16,000 people a year are diagnosed with lupus in the United States and that 1.5 million Americans, or some 5 million people worldwide, have some form of lupus, according to the Centers for Disease Control and Prevention in the United States. In addition, the currently available data suggests that the systemic and discoid forms of lupus together are more common than cystic fibrosis, leukemia, muscular dystrophy, and multiple sclerosis combined.

Lupus chiefly manifests in women between the ages of fifteen and forty-four years old, but it can appear in men and, in fewer cases, children. Overall, it is estimated that 90 percent of the cases diagnosed are women of childbearing age.

For reasons still not entirely understood, people of Native American, African, Hispanic, and Asian descent are more likely to develop lupus than those of Caucasian descent, according to the Lupus Foundation of America as of January 2017. It therefore affects African Americans, Hispanics/Latinos, Alaskan natives, and native Hawaiians and other Pacific Islanders to a greater extent. Some estimates put the likelihood of women of color having lupus at two to three times that of Caucasian women. Furthermore, "patients from minority populations tend to have an acute disease onset, presenting a greater number of and more severe clinical manifestations" but "their causes remain poorly explained" (Uribe and Alarçon 2003). Because it is hard to diagnose, these estimates need to be put in this context. It is possible that as awareness and understanding of the symptoms improves, these statistics may change.

Lupus is not contagious—in other words, you cannot catch it from a sufferer. As already stated, it is classified as an autoimmune condition. This means that when it manifests, a person's immune system becomes overactive and instead of protecting the body from bacteria, viruses, and diseases in a beneficial way, the system goes into overdrive and starts attacking healthy cells as well. Why certain people's immune systems behave in this manner is not fully understood and is a subject for ongoing research. It is thought that environmental, lifestyle, and socioeconomic factors may have influence, but likewise, there are many cases for which currently there is no rhyme or reason.

There is evidence to suggest that there may be a genetic predisposition to lupus and to other autoimmune diseases. Within the family tree, there can be significant and important examples, such as cases of lung disorders, rheumatoid arthritis, Raynaud's syndrome, and skin sensitivities. The likelihood of lupus being diagnosed pre-1960 is also a variable. At the present time, scientists can discover "no clear Mendelian [also known as classic and simple genetics] pattern of inheritance … with siblings of SLE patients having a risk of disease of [only] about 2 [percent]" (Scofield 2015).

External environmental factors and individual sensitivities may be meaningful, particularly when it comes to analyzing why some people have flares and why some are in remission and others are not.

Recent research has also identified that lupus flares can be set in motion by bacterial and viral infections, with the Epstein-Barr virus, which is best known as the cause of mononucleosis, or glandular fever, implicated by some. However, there is also considerable anecdotal evidence of flares being triggered by periods of trauma and acute stress.

The latest research by Dr. Martin Kriegel, who is professor of Immunobiology and Medicine at Yale University, has discovered that when a protein called RO60, which usually protects the tissues of the body in the skin, nose, and guts, comes under attack, it activates an autoimmune response. Dr. Kriegel has concluded that although genes may predispose people to lupus, adverse symptoms are triggered and sustained by bacteria. This is important when it comes to understanding what sets off flares, but it may also bode well for future research into cures because "genes are fixed, but microbes are really malleable" (Kriegel 2018).

Although a low percentage of people with lupus will die prematurely due to complications, primarily because of damage to major organs or infections, "the majority of people living with lupus can now expect to live a normal life span," according to the Lupus Foundation of America, which puts this at 80 percent to 90 percent of those diagnosed. The British Society for Rheumatology notes in its latest guidelines, published in 2017, "Death from active lupus is rare in the UK" (Gordon 2017).

These survival rates are now possible due to ongoing improvements in the recognition and treatment of the disease and to modern drug treatments. Medications for lupus, which I will discuss in detail further on, are all borrowed from other diseases, and a medicine tailored specifically for it has yet to be produced. As we have previously stated, to date there is no complete cure. There are drugs that can control the disease, but their application is a process of experimentation, at the outset and on an ongoing basis. For the majority of patients, the selection, combination, and dosage of their medications are in continuous trial and adjustment as the path of the disease fluctuates.

For some, the symptoms can be considerable and often life changing, particularly during flares, but for others there may be no outward signs at all and the manifestations can be mild. There can also be substantial periods of remission or dormancy, with or without medication. This erratic path is in itself a problem, as the British Society for Rheumatology notes: "The disease is prone to relapses and remissions, resulting in considerable morbidity due to flares of disease activity and accumulated damage" (Gordon 2017).

A survey published late in 2015 analyzed the complete remission of lupus patients over a thirty-two-year period and found that 14.5 percent achieved complete remission for at least three years (Medina-Quiñones 2015). The survey also acknowledged advancements in diagnosis and treatment over the last decade. The latest study, in 2017, which drew on results from 130 clinicians from thirty countries, showed that "up to 17 [percent] of patients with lupus may successfully stop all medications for a period of time" (Ngamjanyaporn 2017). The findings also recognized that 86.9 percent of all clinicians now prescribe hydroxychloroquine, even in cases of only mild symptoms or five-year remissions. In reality, the true benefits of increasing awareness and improved treatments are yet to be fully played out.

Amy's Story

"I always had a bit of a history with fatigue, the odd achy joint, and really bad Raynaud's, but in fact it was the doctors that suggested [lupus] and I was downplaying all my symptoms. I had positive test results but hadn't realized how serious everything was until I had my first flare, and then when I was flaring, everyone believed me: the emergency GP, my tutors in university, my friends/family, and the rheumatologist. I am so lucky to have been surrounded by such sympathetic and understanding people."

This is why it is imperative to continue to raise the profile of lupus in order to ensure that Amy's good experience is increasingly widespread.

The History of Lupus Treatment

The reason the majority of people know little about lupus becomes clear when you look at its medical history. This shows that rapid progress on research and treatment into the condition has only really taken place in the last seventy years or so. The history also helps us to make sense of its strange clinical name and lays the basis for understanding the modern medicines used to treat it. If lupus is a jigsaw, then its history forms the edge pieces of an overall picture.

Accounts of what we know as lupus date as far back as 460 BC, when the famous Greek physician Hippocrates (the origin of the Hippocratic oath, namely "first, do no harm," which is historically taken by doctors) wrote about a severe red facial rash. Indeed, the earliest descriptions of the disease centered on its skin manifestations, with the term *lupus* itself attributed to thirteenth-century physician Rogerius Frugardi of Salerno in Italy, who lived between 1145 and 1195 AD. Salerno had a strong medical tradition, and Rogerius Frugardi wrote his famous medical work the *Practica Chirurgiae*, or, in translation, *The Practice of Surgery*, in about 1170 AD (Roseman 2002). The brilliant Rogerius, going into more detail than Hippocrates, described facial lesions as indented and red, which looked to his mind as if the person had been bitten by a wolf. With the Latin word for wolf being *lupus*, the foundation term for the condition was born.

We then roll forward hundreds of years to the mid-nineteenth century, again with the impact on the skin. The term *erythematosus* was coined by French physician Pierre Cazenave in 1851, who added the Greek word for red or blush, *erythema*, to the Latin *lupus*, hence lupus erythematosus.

In the mid-1800s, two leading Viennese physicians, Ferdinand von Hebra and his son-in-law Moritz Kaposi, studied lupus. At first, Kaposi looked more closely at the lesions and their distribution evenly spread on either side of the nose, and he thought it looked like a pair of wings and therefore described it as looking like a butterfly. Although in practice it is now recognized that a limited percentage of sufferers actually experience the classic butterfly rash, as we have noted earlier, nevertheless a butterfly has become the symbol of many lupus support associations worldwide. It is also often described as a malar rash, from the Latin word *mal* for cheekbone.

Going beyond the skin, Kaposi also wrote for the first time about symptoms extending to other organs of the body. He went on to record evidence that he had found linking the distinctive lesions with physical ailments, including swelling and pain in the small and large joints, lymphatic problems, fever, weight loss, anemia, and general central nervous system involvement. So he and his father-in-law are accredited with being the first to record lupus as responsible for symptoms throughout the body, or behaving "systemically." This led to the final piece of the modern description of the disease being put in place, namely "systemic," now giving us the full modern name systemic lupus erythematosus.

In 1894, Dr. Thomas Payne, a leading physician at St Thomas' Hospital in London, recognized that chloroquine, the antimalarial treatment, might have wider applications for lupus, such as treating the general feelings of fatigue, malaise, and joint pain.

In my mid-teens, I had an invitation from a great school friend to go to her family home in Dubai for the summer holidays, and I had to take anti-malaria tablets. While in Dubai, and for some weeks after my return, I felt amazing, full of energy with no inexplicable bouts of fatigue or aches, and had a wonderful time, with one of my favorite activities being ice-skating on an Olympic-size rink built in the middle of the desert. With hindsight, now it all makes sense, as, unwittingly, for the first time in my life, I had been taking exactly the right medicine to keep my completely unrecognized lupus under control. Furthermore, because it had been simply too hot to go out into the sunshine, at over forty degrees Celsius, almost all our time was spent in the shade or inside with air-conditioning. So while benefitting from the dry desert heat, direct sun exposure did not present a problem. There is more about lupus photosensitivity in due course.

Hydroxychloroquine is derived from quinine and cinchonine, and both were sourced originally from the bark of the cinchona tree, which is native to Peru and used to treat malaria. Romantically, the tree was named after Countess Francisca de Chinchón, who, the story goes, miraculously recovered from a severe feverish illness when given an extract of the bark of a local tree by native healers in the seventeenth century. The legend of the tree bark grew, and its use spread from Latin America to Europe. In 1820, two French chemists named Pierre Joseph Pelletier and Joseph Canentou extracted the quinine in the bark and then distilled and purified it. So effective was the extract against malaria that by the mid-1930s, industrial-sized plantations of the chinchona tree were being grown in Java to meet global demand.

However, the Japanese occupied Java in World War II, so a synthetic version had to be created to protect Allied troops from malaria while fighting in the Pacific. Also during the war, the medicine was found to be beneficial for some of the major symptoms of lupus, namely muscle and joint pain, inflammation in the linings of the lungs and the heart, rashes and fatigue. By 1955, hydroxychloroquine was included in the World Health Organization's List of Essential Medicines, thereby rubber-stamping its effectiveness and safety. The latest thinking is that hydroxychloroquine is also thought to prevent lupus spreading to other organs such as the kidneys and the central nervous system and "may help to reduce flares by as much as 50 [percent]," according to the Johns Hopkins Lupus Centre, who regard it as "key to controlling lupus long-term" and go so far as to call these antimalarials a "sort of lupus life insurance." Johns Hopkins was established in 1876 and was America's first research university and is home to nine world-class academic divisions.

Unfortunately, on returning to temperate England, there was no longer any need for me to take precautions against malaria-carrying mosquitos, and approximately one month after my return, under medical advice, the quinine stopped. How was I—and those around me—to know that this would prove a hugely poor course of action?

Hindsight now allows me to understand the series of events that followed. On the rebound, my body did not appreciate the loss of the antimalarial and began to swell. Mystery edema puffed up my face, eyes, hands, feet, and ankles; and severe stomach cramps began, together with bouts of sudden fatigue. Now I understand that the inflammation in the body caused by lupus "can lead to a buildup of fluids in the abdominal cavity called ascites and symptoms can include severe abdominal pain [and] tenderness" (Lupus UK 2017). Of course, this excess fluid came back many years later, in 2012, when, together with my high fever, it led once again to my admission to the hospital. Clearly it is a distinctive symptom of the way that my lupus manifests.

Back in the 1980s, having undergone tests at my local general practice, conclusions ranged from the edema being diagnosed as "mere puppy fat" by one doctor, to another more accurately stating that a set of blood tests showed "some kind of autoimmune reaction." Another diagnosed "idiopathic edema." Delighted by the news that my symptoms were the result of something that sounded conclusive, my euphoria was short-lived when I looked it up, and I remember that this took some effort because it was pre-Internet and Google. I found that *idiopathic* stemmed from the Greek and meant "one's own disease," or an illness not connected to any particular cause—in other words, "not understood." Therefore, I was pretty much back in the dark.

Nevertheless, my general practitioner at the time designated the swelling to be the result of water retention and prescribed strong diuretics to eliminate the fluid. The diuretics had the side effect of lowering my blood pressure so dramatically that I would faint suddenly, without warning, and against this background, I studied for and sat for A and S levels in the UK and prepared for university.

It would then take almost thirty years for my lupus to be correctly diagnosed. This gives me firsthand appreciation of the importance of broadening the recognition of lupus, understanding that in the early 1980s, the chances of my being correctly diagnosed were extremely slim; indeed, it would have been leading edge at the time. I wondered how different could things have been if I had instead been given continuing treatment with my "lupus life insurance" of antimalarials.

<u>Coco's Story</u>

"Back in the twentieth century, few of us had ever heard of these categories of illness [autoimmune conditions] ... and of course, back then, there was no Internet to aid research. ... When my lupus was finally diagnosed in 2011, I was 90 percent housebound. I joined Lupus UK and began to learn about lupus. Before long, I realized my experience of lifestyle management could probably help others on our UK forum, which made all those decades of suffering seem almost worthwhile. Also, if there was anything I could do to help others like me feel less lost and alone, I simply had to do it."

Between 1895 and 1903, Canadian physician Sir William Osler carried out further groundbreaking research into the systemic nature of lupus, and crucially he noted that lupus could go into periods of remission before becoming active again. So he was the first to identify a hallmark of systemic lupus, namely the flare.

Having taken my A levels and having a place at university confirmed,

I fainted once so deeply after an evening of severe stomach cramps that I hyperventilated, and as I struggled for breath, my distressed family called an ambulance. At accident and emergency, my ability to ease off the bed, hold tightly onto my father's arm, and walk shakily along a white line on the floor deemed me fit for discharge, with no further investigation. I recall going in and out of consciousness on the way home in the car. I then spent days resting either in bed or in an easy chair "looking like a little old woman," David, a work colleague, commented. In retrospect, it is easy to identify a classic lupus flare, but at the time, no one knew what was wrong with me and the family referred to me as "fragile."

You can see from the geographic spread of the physicians who made it part of their life's work to identify and classify lupus that this is a global disease. It was not until the mid-twentieth century, when strides in diagnosis and treatment started to be made, that doctors began to save the lives of patients suffering from the more severe forms of the condition. Sufferers previously could have limited life expectancy and just fade away as the lupus spread systemically through the body until it reached and destroyed key organs. The Lupus Foundation of America notes that in 1955, only 50 percent of people diagnosed with severe lupus were expected to live more than four years, but by 1969, that figure had extended to ten years.

In 1941, Dr. Paul Klemperer, leading a team at Mount Sinai Hospital in New York, wrote in-depth pathological descriptions of lupus, devising the term "collagen disease." This became the foundation of the modern categorization of lupus as an "autoimmune" disorder and is the start of the appreciation that lupus is one of a group of diseases that adversely impact the immune system. Klemperer understood that in these cases, the immune system becomes overactive and turns on itself, attacking healthy cells and damaging its own tissues. Then, instead of fighting off external diseases, the immune deficiency also causes vulnerability to infections.

The year 1948 saw the breakthrough discovery of the LE (lupus erythematosus) cell by Dr. Malcolm Hargreaves and associates Helen Morton and Dr. Robert Morton at the famous Mayo Clinic in Scottsdale, Arizona. Crucially, this discovery allowed the presence of lupus to be identified pathologically—in other words, by a straightforward blood test.

In 1949, also at the Mayo, Dr. Philip Hench used a recently discovered hormone called cortisone, which was proving beneficial in the treatment of rheumatoid arthritis to treat lupus patients, and it "immediately showed a dramatic ability to save lives" (Lupus UK 2018). Dr. Hench was awarded the Nobel Prize in Medicine for the discovery of applications for corticosteroids, and lupus was one of the first conditions that he trialed, with results that could be nothing short of miraculous.

Two other immunological markers were discovered in the 1950s as being hallmarks of lupus, leading to the recognition that people suffering from lupus had antinuclear antibodies in their blood. This allowed doctors to directly test for the presence of these antibodies. Further research showed that lupus patients also had other antibodies present, some of which attached themselves to patients' DNA. This ultimately led to anti-DNA tests that proved very useful in tying down the presence of the disease. This test is included in a suite of blood tests, as previously illustrated, that are used in modern medicine to conclude an official diagnosis.

Antiphospholipid antibodies had been identified and researched in the 1940s and were known to include the lupus anticoagulant and a false-positive test for syphilis—and that the two were linked. However, it was not until the 1980s that a research group under the aegis of Professor Graham Hughes began to explore the link in greater detail. Professor Hughes now works out of the London Lupus Centre.

A researcher within the Hughes team, Nigel Harris, then found that cardiolipin, an antiphospholipid antibody, was the reason for a link between lupus and syphilis. He found that the syphilis test detects the presence of an antibody called reagin, but reagin reacts to cardiolipin, so those giving false-positive syphilis tests actually had cardiolipin antibodies in their blood. Patients with syphilis would have cardiolipin but would not have lupus. Patients with lupus were also likely to test positive for the lupus anticoagulant and other lupus tests. Harris developed a specific test to identify the presence of cardiolipin, but he also realized that the presence of these antiphospholipid antibodies were, importantly, associated with an increased likelihood of blood clots.

Others in the Hughes laboratory then went onto explore the link further. Antiphospholipid syndrome (APS) is now more commonly known as Hughes syndrome, and the finding was published in 1983. They found that people who have systemic lupus erythematosus are at increased risk of having Hughes syndrome, but some do not, myself included, having been tested for it by one of Professor Hughes's team. Indeed, it is recognized that it is actually more common for Hughes syndrome to exist outside of lupus. There are in fact two kinds of antiphospholipid syndrome, and it is the secondary form that develops alongside another autoimmune disorder; this is usually lupus.

Hughes syndrome influences the blood and its ability to clot correctly, and it can manifest in any organ, creating potentially fatal conditions such as heart attacks and strokes, but also headaches and depression. Migraines, in addition to being triggered by photosensitivity, as previously examined, can also be the result of antiphospholipid syndrome. Recognition is crucial in pregnancy, where its presence causes miscarriages, stillbirths, and other complications such as preeclampsia. The excellent news is that, if identified, the London Lupus Centre currently describes Hughes syndrome as "highly treatable ... with often a dramatic improvement."

You can now see from the history that recognition of the general impact of lupus on the body only started to be recorded in the middle of the eighteenth century, while modern drug treatment with antimalarials was then discovered right at the end of the nineteenth century. Life-saving tests and cortisone drugs then emerged in the mid-twentieth century, with further critical research concluded at the end of the twentieth century.

Modern Treatments

For clarity, it is valuable to describe the core modern medications now used to treat and control the main symptoms of systemic lupus erythematosus. The forums are often dominated by medication queries—some are generic, others highly individual. In addition, because there are often comorbid conditions and complications, as has been recognized, many will require other treatments, and it is common for repeat prescription printouts for those diagnosed in the UK to run to three pages or more. Nevertheless, with the aim of giving a broad understanding in layman's language, these are understood to be the leading medications for systemic lupus erythematosus at this time. They are ranked below, starting with the lowest potency and possible side effects, ascending to those prescribed as the lupus symptoms worsen.

Aspirin

This is traditionally used to reduce fever, mild to moderate pain, and swelling, but it can cause stomach ulceration in some patients. Therefore, in some cases it may be replaced by non-steroidal medications that are more modern. As it is also known to prevent heart attacks and strokes, it is often prescribed as a cornerstone treatment for lupus.

Acetaminophen

Paracetamol can be acquired over the counter in the United States, under brand names such as Tylenol, to control pain and reduce fever, and it is often used in conjunction with other medications. It may have less adverse effects on the stomach than prescription medicines, but it can cause liver and kidney problems, so the correct dosage, especially if you have lupus nephritis, should be discussed with your doctor.

Modern Non-Steroidals (NSAIDs)

Ibuprofen, naproxen, diclofenac, and celecoxib are widely used to reduce pain, bring down temperatures, and reduce swelling. They go under a whole range of trade names, including Motrin, Advil, Neurofen, Naprosyn, Voltarol, and Celebrex. Their suitability in terms of relief and side effects can vary from patient to patient, and they are often applied on a trial-and-error basis according to guidance on their website from the London Lupus Centre. Side effects include nausea, stomach upset, and even ulcers; they may also interfere with the function of the kidneys. Patients may also find that they bruise more easily.

Antimalarials

These are hydroxychloroquine, chloroquine phosphate, and quinacrine. As we explored earlier when looking at the history of lupus, these were originally used to treat malaria. They were found to improve pain in the muscles and joints, rashes, mouth sores, fatigue, fever, and inflammation of the linings of the heart and the lungs. Their use in patients with lupus is becoming more common, and one recent study found that over 50 percent of patients with systemic lupus erythematosus were prescribed hydroxychloroquine (HCQ), reinforced by the LUMINA study that confirmed "clear survival benefit of HCQ therapy in patients with SLE" (Alarçon 2007).

It has also been discovered that a possible side effect of prolonged high-dose treatment with hydroxychloroquine has a negative impact on the eyes, with deposition of the drug into the cornea. According to the Royal College of Ophthalmologists in the UK for the worst-case scenarios: "In some people with more advanced retinopathy, stopping hydroxychloroquine treatment does not stop the condition from getting worse. At the moment, there is no treatment for hydroxychloroquine toxicity." The very latest research published in 2017 concluded the following: "Hydroxychloroquine retinal toxicity is far more common than previously considered: an overall prevalence of 7.5 [percent] was identified in patients taking HCQ for more than five years, rising to almost 20 [percent] after twenty years of treatment" (Yusuf 2017). This has led to newly released guidelines by the National Health Service (NHS) in the UK in 2018 for those on hydroxychloroquine long term, for regular eye screening and guidance, also for low doses of between two to four hundred milligrams daily for adults.

<u>Corticosteroids</u>

These are hydrocortisone, prednisolone, methylprednisolone, and dexamethasone. These vary in strength. Hydrocortisone is weaker than prednisolone, methylprednisolone is stronger, and dexamethasone is very potent. Corticosteroids control inflammation and regulate the immune system, which in turn suppresses lupus symptoms. Corticosteroids can be applied topically, taken orally, and given intravenously, the latter in severe cases. Since they were first applied with lifesaving and miraculous benefits in the late 1940s, short-term side effects, including an increase in weight, indigestion, and muscle weakness have been identified. Prednisolone is a synthetic form of the hormone cortisol, which is normally produced by the adrenal gland. Production of cortisol increases in stressful situations, and it stimulates the appetite and redirects the accumulation of fat. As a result, it can cause weight gain, in particular around the waist, the bottom half of the face (referred to as corticosteroid moon face), and the neck.

Undoubtedly, these symptoms are now more widely recognized, as are the potential long-term problems of high-level doses, such as the softening of bones, the occasional breakage of bones, and thinning of the blood. Because of this increased understanding, you will usually be required to have a DEXA (dual-energy x-ray absorptiometry) bone density scan to reassure your doctors that your bones have not been damaged by a period of high corticosteroid medication. According to research (Jehle 2003), patients deemed to be at risk are those taking more than 30mg of hydrocortisone or 7.5mg of prednisolone for extended periods.

Great care is now given to administer larger doses for the shortest time possible and to wean patients off corticosteroids as soon as it is practical or to have the long-term maintenance dosages in the low single digits. Support for the bones in the form of calcium and vitamin D supplements is also standard procedure.

It is now recognized that corticosteroids can have mental implications too, including lack of concentration, agitation, anxiety, paranoia, and insomnia. A December 2013 study recorded "sleep disorders characterized by restlessness and insomnia in 73 [percent] of cases" (Ciriaco 2013), while withdrawal from higher doses has also been shown in some cases to promote mood swings and depression. Ciriaco and colleagues concluded that 1 percent of patients taking a dose higher than forty milligrams will have an adverse psychological reaction, and at eighty milligrams, this increases to 18.4 [percent] (Ciriaco 2013). After conversations with fellow corticosteroid takers and given my own experience of the alternative, deeply calm energy achieved with breath work, mindfulness, and transcendental meditation, these drugs activate a "wired" energy in the body and the mind. They create a feeling of agitation that is unsettling and tends to heighten any other feelings of anxiety, irritation, or insecurity.

Stomach Liners

Taking corticosteroids can irritate the stomach, especially if taking higher doses. This is why it is recommended that tablets be taken with food or milk, but you may also be prescribed a liner in the form of ranitidine hydrochloride or omeprazole to prevent heartburn, nausea, and/or vomiting.

<u>Codeine Phosphate</u>

This opioid prescription medication is given for pain that is not cured by NSAIDs; it can cause drowsiness, confusion, and depression. It is part of a group including hydrocodone and oxycodone, which are generally not first-line treatments because they are addictive. It should never be taken with alcohol.

<u>Immunosuppressants</u>

In more severe cases, where the previous drugs are not controlling the lupus and it is the result of an overactive immune system, these medications are prescribed to try to bring the condition under control, particularly if the patients have active kidney disease or are not responding sufficiently well to corticosteroids. These usually take the form of azathioprine, cyclosporine, and methotrexate, although there are others. As these drugs reduce the formation of blood in the bone marrow, regular monitoring with blood tests is considered essential.

Taking them can increase susceptibility to small infections such as those in the eyes, throat, and nails. Given the problems with extremities amongst lupus patients who already have Raynaud's and peripheral neuropathy (nerve damage), it is wise to take extra care of your hands and feet in general. You may need a good chiropodist, and if you are having manicures, remain alert to the hygiene of used emery boards, for example.

Elsewhere, an annual flu jab is usually considered essential, and lupus patients are specifically advised to avoid exposure to the herpes varicella virus in the form of shingles or chicken pox. Signs of shingles are a band of pain followed by a red blotchy rash that develops into itchy blisters. Common sites are the chest, abdomen, or upper face. If you do get shingles when on immunosuppressants, then you are advised to contact your doctor straightaway so that you can be given antiviral medication immediately and monitored for complications.

Patients with moderate and severe lupus on immunosuppressants have to be careful of infection in general, with extra care on basic hygiene such as handwashing and antibacterial wipes for public spaces. It may also be necessary to reschedule any visitors with infections or viruses.

<u>Morphine Sulfate</u>

The opioid painkiller is prescribed to alleviate severe and chronic pain not cured by other lesser forms of relief. It can cause extreme drowsiness, and you are advised not to drive or use machinery while on morphine, as it has a narcoleptic quality. It is also recognized as being highly addictive.

<u>Newer Medicines</u>

In recent years, mycophenolate mofetil, previously given to prevent organ rejection in transplants, has been increasingly used in lupus, particularly if there is the coexistence of a kidney condition. I will later talk more about my personal experience of this treatment.

In addition, so-called anti-B cell agents, rituximab, and belimunab are now being used internationally in some cases of very severe lupus, although cost can be a factor here.

This list is not intended to replace the comprehensive advice on side effects that is given by the leaflets that accompany both over-the-counter drugs and prescription medicines. It is designed to inform you about the most common medicines prescribed, their major possible difficulties, and how they are used with mild, moderate, and severe lupus.

The modern approach is to use high doses only when necessary and for the shortest possible time and to increase and decrease amounts in line with disease activity or flares. The ultimate goal is remission, with low-maintenance doses of aspirin and hydroxychloroquine as well as paracetamol or NSAIDs for intermittent aches and pains. If hydroxychloroquine cannot be tolerated, which it can in the majority of cases, it can be replaced with mepacrine, which can have the side effect of turning the skin slightly golden yellow.

In cases of moderate and severe lupus, rheumatologists may layer treatments from mild through to the more aggressive in order to get very active periods or severe flares under control. Regular monitoring with blood tests and scans is standard procedure. Although differing levels of success may be achieved with different drugs, this may not be sustained and a change may be required. Layering and experimentation are in fact the norm for a set of medications that, as previously stated, are ultimately all borrowed from elsewhere, with a groundbreaking medication specifically designed to cure lupus and/or other autoimmune conditions yet to be found. Shinya Yamaka noted, "I think that in the twenty-first century, medical biology will advance at a more rapid pace than before," and many live in hope that this will be the case for the treatment of lupus.

So in line with the brilliant research of the last two hundred years and having been officially diagnosed, to my immense relief, prescriptions were issued for a high dose of corticosteroids to be taken orally, the stomach liner omeprazole to protect against the problems associated with the high dose of corticosteroids, and pain relief in the form of diclofenac.

By a stroke of luck, the major rooms in my house were all on the ground floor, including the main bedroom, as stairs were impossible for me. Weak and in constant pain, I waited for the medicines to work their magic. You go to the doctors, you are diagnosed and they prescribe the right medicine, and you get better, right? Well, it's not so fast and not so simple. Within a few days, it became clear that matters were not going according to plan—in fact, definitely not going right at all!

The natural progression of the disease, for all those years unrecognized and untreated, combined with the severe infection that had me hospitalized, had actually sparked a most damaging flare indeed. Far from this being the end of my problems, the next few weeks would see me instead spiral rapidly downward into a morass of acute symptoms. These would leave me a husk of my former self, who, in the words of my London consultant, would "fade fast" toward a life-threatening state as the fallout from the flare crashed through my body.

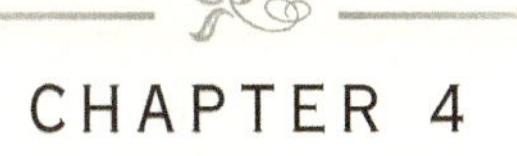

CHAPTER 4

The Physical Symptoms

*Our patients never feel well. They have pain
and fatigue that cannot be described.*
—Dr. Michelle Petri, Johns Hopkins Lupus Center

So far, we have defined the official diagnosis, the history, and the core medicines that anchor a basic understanding of this complex condition. Nevertheless, what is also evident from studying the forums and blogs over the last six years is that the day-to-day reality of living with lupus is still confusing to many. Although they do not appear on the official diagnostic list, there is a battery of associated symptoms indicative of lupus. I have learned the hard way that these are often unacknowledged or massively understated, leaving patients, their loved ones, and supporters in a no-man's-land of uncertainty and self-doubt. Therefore, it is enormously valuable to dispel this confusion and to describe these and their true impact. The two front-runners leading out this pack of typical but unofficial symptoms are pain and fatigue.

Pain

Three days after leaving the hospital, I reacted to the high dose of corticosteroids and made an emergency phone call to my consultant's secretary, saying, "My insides feel as if they have been napalmed."

The dramatic use of a Vietnam War reference to describe the acute burning sensation tearing down through my chest and into my stomach led to my corticosteroid dose being reduced, which solved one problem but created another: my most pressing problem became pain.

In a survey by Lupus UK, 65 percent of respondents listed pain as the most difficult aspect of lupus, with some form of 24-7 pain not being unusual. The Lupus Foundation of America reported that over 90 percent of lupus patients would experience joint or muscle pain during the course of their illness, especially during periods of increased disease activity.

Pain gripped all my major joints, shoulders, elbows, knees, and occasionally my hips—also, strangely, the base of my thumbs. My legs were swollen and red, especially around the knees, which could almost double in size, and the main veins bulged lividly. Small patches of red and purple spider veins emerged, and I gazed down with astonishment at limbs that had transformed from smooth and beach-ready into those of a very old woman in a matter of days. Tenderness and soreness in the joints would rapidly escalate through burning and throbbing to an unbearable ache along the connecting muscles, giving the sensation of entire limb pain. Intense, stabbing pain could also grip certain muscles selectively. My arms were very bad; my legs were worse.

Furthermore, the unrelenting pain piled on the exhaustion. Nights were increasingly difficult because unresolved pain woke me every two hours. Unable to get consistent comfort or rest in any position, although propped up high on several pillows with my legs raised, I would shake for an hour at a time. A selection of soft, supportive pillows moved with me from the bed to the sofa and back again. My heavy body grew increasingly stiff and rigid such that, trying to maintain a sense of humor, I called myself the Tin Man, from *The Wizard of Oz*. Stiff fingers curled inward to the palms of my hands, and stumbling between rooms, I held them out in front of me like little claws.

None of the mind-body techniques learned later (and covered in part II) were then at my disposal, and as the days advanced, the grim truth began to dawn that the corticosteroids were taking their time to have any impact and the diclofenac prescription was simply not up to the task. This resulted in my lurching in and out of severe pain, and as time went on, it became evident that the pain was largely uncontrolled and escalating.

A fortnight after leaving the hospital, it was a bank holiday weekend in the UK. Unable to rest or sleep properly for days, I had become exhausted and that night prowled the house for hours, unable to get relief, shaking and rigid with distress. Around midnight, I discovered some herbal arnica gel in the medicine cupboard, and it seemed like a good option to try spreading that up and down my arms to try to calm the burning, throbbing sensation there at least.

That did not work, and half an hour later, raiding the medicine cupboard again, I applied ibuprofen gel, adding to the diclofenac already in the system. That did not work either, and it seemed impracticable to treat legs and hips the same way. One o'clock … two o'clock … moving between the sofa and the kitchen so as not to disturb the rest of the sleeping family. Finally, by four in the morning, at the end of my tether, I woke my husband, begging for help. With the understanding of over two decades together, he did not question the level of crisis.

Early in the morning on a bank holiday, it seemed an impossible task to achieve a rescue, but remarkably, a doctor came out to see me, reaching us some hour and a half later. He found a trembling huddle on a sofa. My gratitude for his instant recognition of my predicament, his compassion, and his kind words remain with me to this day. "My dear lady" he said calmly as he clicked open his black case, "you do not need to be in this much pain."

With my permission as the dawn broke, he injected me with morphine sulfate, an opioid painkiller. With immense gratitude, I slept for seven hours straight on the sofa, the limbs relaxed and the pain finally under control.

Now I understand that I had suffered what is referred to as a bout of breakthrough pain, where if the underlying pain is not adequately controlled, then a patient can experience an intense spike. In this situation, modern fast-acting narcotics can provide relief.

The doctor left me a prescription for a low dose of morphine sulfate in oral solution so that I could better manage my limb pain and treat such sharp escalations. Understandably, there is a great deal of concern about escalating dependency and addiction in America and the UK, indeed worldwide, to opioid painkillers. Dependency can occur rapidly, and if fueled by applications for prescriptions from multiple sources or even an escalation to their illegal acquisition, then the relationship is clearly out of control. It is not the aim of this book to discuss this complicated and challenging area, beyond appreciating the addictive dangers of these medications and to add a warning along with other louder and louder voices. I must clarify that if you find yourself crossing the line of exceeding your original prescription, and especially if you start to look for alternative sources to add to your original doctor's prescription, then there is no doubt that you should seek immediate professional advice and help.

It is the aim of this book to describe my journey from a purely medical approach to how I used holistic techniques to do the following:

- Much more effectively control pain in combination with prescribed pain relief
- Reduce the severity and duration of escalating pain and breakout pain
- Eliminate tolerance to prescribed pain relief, tolerance being where the body adjusts the need for the drugs upward to achieve the same level of pain relief
- Gradually reduce the dosage and dependence on medical pain relief

In the second and third parts of this book, I will demonstrate how these goals were achieved.

According to my doctors, the dose of morphine sulfate in oral solution prescribed was relatively low, but it had my immense gratitude for the new level of control that it gave me over escalating pain. Taken as and when needed, it gave me the option of phasing in relief as I experienced fluctuations throughout the day and night. Nonetheless, the pain remained constant.

Concerned about my ongoing pain, my doctors and community nurses were keen to eliminate it completely with stronger drugs and/or different delivery systems. On the suggestion of my general practitioners, one of whom is a pain specialist and the doctor at the college for severely disabled students at which I had counselled, giving me firsthand knowledge of the severity and complexity of the pain conditions handled by him on a daily basis, I trialed transdermal patches, including fentanyl. Fentanyl is eighty to one hundred times more potent than morphine and many times that of heroin, and it left me feeling so drugged and without any periods of lucidity that many other functions were impossible. Yes, my pain was gone, but it left me semicomatose.

A level down to morphine patches was also trialed, on a similar principle, trying to iron out the peaks and the troughs and ideally eliminate the continuous pain. It once again left me out of it all the time, and anything approaching daily life was unfeasible. Taking the oral solution at least allowed me to calibrate precisely the amount needed so I could take it to suit the range of pain as it changed, with support from the nonaddictive diclofenac. This method became the best that could be achieved for me, but having spoken to fellow lupus patients, it is clear that pain is highly personal and you have to find a system that fits you. Unfortunately, this can be a process of elimination that is reliant on a helpful and flexible medical team supporting you. You may need to persevere to find a solution that best manages your disease profile and your level of activity.

Getting out of bed became the first major challenge of the day. On waking, I would be so stiff that my limbs needed to be unbent gradually and then my whole body eased out from under the covers and onto the floor. "Our first steps in the morning call on two hundred pulling muscles" (Knaster 1996). This could be so unbelievably difficult that one morning it struck me that one way to avoid the painful untangling, or at the very least to speed it up, would be to drop down from the bed onto the floor in one quick movement. Mulling over the plan for what must have been at least ten minutes, weighing up the agony of unravelling versus the attraction of a swift resolution, eventually the swift option won. Having fallen on the carpet, the realization hit that I was far too weak and it was going to be too painful for me to get up unaided. I had to cry out for help. What can I say—pain really messes with your judgment!

Washing became an excruciating and exhausting daily routine, with a seat required in and right outside the shower to rest on. One day I felt it necessary to lie down after the shower, only to wake up on the bed two and half hours later wrapped in my dressing gown because the whole process had proved so draining.

Controlling the pain became my number one priority. This outranked all other considerations, as untrammeled, it could leave me writhing on the bed or sofa, much to the distress of my husband and my dogs. Without the pain under control, no other functions were possible. There would be brief windows when it would ease down but then just a matter of time before it would return with force, heading toward me like a large truck at a high speed.

My biggest problem, as identified by the community nurses who came to look after me in pain crises, was my tendency to tough out the pain for too long. Their advice was to be in front of the pain and take enough pain relief ahead of an escalation. Stoicism was the wrong approach, and it was better to act sooner rather than later or suffer the consequences. "Please take enough medication and front run the pain, Karen," they would say in exasperated tones.

Despite now having improved relief, my reality was that the pain, weakness, and fatigue were utterly debilitating. Usually too weak to perform even the simplest tasks, my body felt completely alien. Previously relied upon to go where my head had led, biddable and totally taken for granted, it had morphed into an entity that had to be micromanaged with the greatest possible care, and even then it could be mercurial. My body had developed a personality of its own, whose tantrums were pain and its moods exhaustion.

Fatigue

Research estimates that as many as 91 percent of people with lupus experience fatigue as one of the main symptoms, and many patients find that they have to manage their activities with immense care to prevent them feeling utterly drained some hours later or the day after. This is known as payback fatigue, and it often poses a recurrent and largely unsolvable problem for lupus patients.

<u>Eliza's Story</u>

"I returned from a skiing trip with severe pain all down both arms and went to see my family doctor on my return to explain my extreme fatigue. I told her that I felt so exhausted that I could literally lie down underneath her desk right then … and fall asleep. Thankfully, my GP knew the family well and that we only ever went to the doctor when something was really, really wrong."

Blood tests went on to confirm a diagnosis of systemic lupus erythematosus. Eliza describes the lupus fatigue that despite medication and careful lifestyle management still catches up with her as feeling "like I am walking through heavy sludge," and she comments that she often feels "like a zombie" with fatigue, while social events can leave her "utterly drained."

Feverishness

A low-grade fever not exceeding 102 degrees Fahrenheit, or some 39 degrees Celsius, is a hallmark of lupus flares, although it can often be masked by substantial doses of aspirin, nonsteroidal anti-inflammatories, and corticosteroids. It can manifest as feeling hot but also as bouts of shaking or shivering fits, what used to be known in older English terms as *ague*. Successive cold and sweating spells followed by pain in the limbs and joints used to be indicative of malaria, so it is perhaps not surprising that those early pioneers made the link and decided to treat lupus with the same medication. My solution is layers of breathable, natural fiber clothing—so cottons, linens, and, more unusually, bamboo, together with an assortment of wraps and rugs. During bouts of fever, usually accompanied in my case with severe pain and nausea, clothing can often be changed in relays.

Lupus Fog

Fighting the pain and fatigue took its toll on my strength, and my functionality was further impaired by the narcoleptic effects, or extreme daytime sleepiness, often with sudden onset, of the morphine sulfate. Lupus patients can experience problems with their concentration, ability to verbalize their thoughts, and remembering things. Reactions may also be slower, either mentally or physically, such as hand-eye coordination. These factors are often referred to collectively as "lupus fog," which can be temporary but recurrent and much worse during flares.

Cognitive reactions may be slowed, making it difficult to absorb information and to multitask as usual. Foggy periods can be incredibly frustrating for patients and for those caring for them as they struggle to articulate their thoughts. Appointments are forgotten, even though there is only one in the diary that day or even that week, and everyday items are misplaced. Pain medications can also cause chemical changes in the brain that can adversely influence cognitive functions, learning ability, and memory.

In one instance, clouded by pain and fatigue, I mistakenly took the wrong small white tablets instead of my corticosteroids for three days in a row and ended up such a moaning, writhing mess that my husband kept track of my tablets for years afterward. He remains vigilant to ensure an adequate supply of pain relief in the house to avoid repeating the experience. For those "foggy" mornings, I keep a list of my medications handy so that I can check them off one by one, and I rely on family and friends to finish my sentences for me when I become stuck halfway through.

The good thing about lupus fog is that it does not usually get progressively worse like Alzheimer's disease or dementia; rather, it is now recognized that lupus cognitive dysfunction is a lower level of central nervous system (CNS) involvement, and as we have stated, referral to a neurologist is common. In rarer instances, if dizziness or headaches start to escalate severely, then it is essential to get them checked out medically because, at worst, CNS involvement can cause strokes and seizures. Although recovering from CNS spikes can be slow, requiring months rather than weeks, the "prognosis is quite good" (Hellman 2011). Nonetheless, it can prove a devastatingly difficult aspect of the disease when it disrupts balance and creates vision problems or leads to behavioral changes.

Nausea

Mismanaging the pain resulted in one uncontrollable outcome for me, harking back to the decision to reduce my pain relief solely to paracetamol when in the hospital: it induced nausea. Well, nothing had changed, and my community nurses informed me that paramedics consider vomiting an indicator of very severe pain. Gastrointestinal sensitivity or central nervous system involvement may also be factors in some lupus patients. When my pain escalated, the nausea hit. This not only prevented me from taking essential medication such as corticosteroids but also, once started despite oral antiemetics, would sometimes not stop without an injected antiemetic.

Initially administered by a local doctor on emergency call-out to prevent admission to the hospital and connection to a drip, subsequently the job became that of local community nurses. Then, following a National Health

Service (NHS) reorganization, which meant that the community nurses could do routine visits but were no longer able to respond to emergency situations, the nurses at my local general practice taught me how to self-inject into my thigh, demonstrating on an orange! Being able to self-inject gives me even more control over my unpredictable condition, but I do miss the compassion and reassurance of the community nurses.

Esophageal Complications

My throat became inflamed and closed in, causing me great difficulty swallowing. This became so bad that I thought choking the most likely cause of my demise rather than any of the other awful symptoms plaguing me. Drinking through straws became a necessity.

The ascites, excess fluid on the stomach, came back twice, requiring admission to the hospital each time to drain the excess, and combined with my problems swallowing and regular nausea from the pain, it resulted in my weight steadily beginning to decline. Eventually, it fell by over two stones (twenty-eight pounds, or slightly under thirteen kilos) to a low of slightly above six stones (eighty-four pounds, or thirty-eight kilos). It is said that leading New York socialites in the 1980s had a motto that "you can never be too rich or too thin," but believe me, you really can lose too much weight, and my close neighbor and good friend Lisa told me subsequently, "It was really not a good look, Karen."

All my curves disappeared, leaving me feeling deeply unfeminine and my stomach concaved and stretched between jutting hip bones. Now I not only felt incredibly frail but looked it too. I sensed alarm when visitors first saw me and could tell that those closest to me were frightened.

Concerned by the weight loss, my doctors referred me to dietitians who prescribed high-calorie drinks to build me back up. These tasted truly awful, with highly artificial flavorings jarring on a palate more used to whole foods. My local general practitioner kindly explained that the calories in these drinks are based on milk, so another way to get the calories in was via full-fat milk and cream. Unable to stomach the greasiness of full-fat milk, organic semi-skimmed became the compromise. If I could swallow nothing else, and primarily to alleviate the look of intense concern on my husband's face, there was always organic vanilla ice cream or Greek yogurt with honey, both of which slipped down easily. Otherwise, a diet of soup, soft fruit, smoothies, juices, and vegetables became my staple, with tomato, avocado, and mozzarella salad a favorite on a good day.

At the time, I could get no clarification as to whether the ascites and the swallow were lupus symptoms or the side effects of medications. In fact, on my hospital visits, medical staff even suggested to me that there might be a psychological element to my not eating, which could be corrected "if I really wanted to eat."

Once again, in the absence of the wider understanding of lupus symptoms, those in authority were holding a psychological cause culprit. Subsequently, on a lupus message board, I found a contributor who had commented that her throat was so swollen and painful that she was hardly able to swallow. Like me, she was wondering whether it was a lupus symptom.

Many other posts and research have since confirmed that esophageal problems are in fact quite usual for lupus. Under the heading "Esophageal Disorders in Lupus," the National Resource Center for Lupus notes, "People with lupus may experience problems in any area of the gastrointestinal tract." They go on to clarify that "when Lupus causes inflammation in the esophagus, stomach acid can back up [and] persistent reflux is known as gastroesophageal reflux disease (GERD) … In addition to reflux, oesophageal problems may also cause difficulty swallowing, a condition called dysphagia." Clearly, I had been suffering from dysphagia. Note that this can reappear along with other symptoms, such as pain and feverishness. At the time, without concrete reassurance of what is in fact a standard symptom, I was instead left full of self-doubt and disempowerment. One of the aims of this book is to prevent you from feeling confused and uncertain, as I did, and to provide you with some ammunition to challenge this psychological diagnosis, should you ever encounter it.

Hair Loss

To add insult to injury, clumps of my hair started to come off on my brush. In answer to my direct question, my London consultant seemed dismissive of my concern and could not confirm whether the hair loss was a result of the lupus or the medication. He instead stated, "Hair loss for someone who has been as sick as you is not unusual," and he gave me a small dismissive flick of his hand.

Subsequently, my research has confirmed that 50 percent of all lupus suffers will experience some form of hair loss either as hair thinning on the scalp or with the loss of eyelashes, eyebrows, beard, and/or body hair. In the case of systemic lupus, the technical description for this symptom is "non-scarring alopecia" (Howard 2017). I can confirm that over time the hair does regrow, and I helped it along with some high-quality tonics applied topically.

The exception to regrowth can be in the case of severe discoid lupus, where lesions on the scalp may cause permanent hair loss. The advice is to get treatment as soon as possible to avoid the lesions establishing. Some hair loss may also be a side effect of medications used to treat lupus, such as antimalarials, corticosteroids, methotrexate, leflunomide, and cyclophosphamide. Again, the advice is to act promptly.

Circadian Rhythms and Barometric Pressure Susceptibility

A word that comes up a lot to describe lupus-targeted joints is *achy*. In my own experience, swelling could appear for no apparent reason and could go up one day and down the next. Disconcertingly, I have watched my thumb joints visibly swell up in front of my eyes for no apparent reason. Similarly, my knees can be super swollen one day and go down two days later, and in classic lupus fashion, one side can increase independent of the other. Furthermore, pain can flit from one joint to another, from the right thumb joint over to the left, within the space of twenty minutes. Peaks and troughs in energy levels accompany this variability, with fatigue often echoing the swelling and pain in the body. Both sets of symptoms can vary according to the time of day, with a consensus that pain and fatigue can get worse as the day goes on. The words "I am much better in the mornings" has been repeated to me numerous times.

Being British, you might expect me to find some way to talk about the weather, but there is indeed a great deal of anecdotal evidence to suggest that joints can react badly to sudden changes in barometric pressure, with the fluid around the joints adversely impacted by shifts to damp and rainy weather and ahead of stormy conditions. The research into the phenomena is less conclusive, with one study finding that pain scores worsened "by one point for each 10 [percent] rise in humidity," but for a change to be clinically relevant, the score needs to be altered by at least ten points. Nonetheless, as Desirée Dorleijn, of the Erasmus University Medical Centre in Rotterdam, who led the research, is reported as saying, "Just because findings didn't reach statistical significance from a researcher's point of view, they can be significant from the patient's point of view" (Jegtvig 2014).

Skin Sensitivity

It is also worth noting that lupus sufferers have a general tendency for sensitive skin, aside from photosensitivity. Therefore, they can have adverse reactions to anything from perfumes to household chemicals. I know that I am highly allergic to some products, including ones marked "organic" or "pure," and from experience, I know that it is wise to try out any new skin care, hair care, and makeup products before using them more widely. This sensitivity also applies to taking extra care with new washing powders, fabric softeners, air fresheners, and household cleaning solutions.

Given this level of sensitivity, mineral-based sunscreens (containing only two ingredients, namely titanium dioxide and zinc oxide) may also be better choices than chemical-based sunscreens, which commonly contain ingredients such as avobenzone, oxybenzone, octinoxate, and octisalate. Mineral-based screens therefore pose less risk, while chemical or synthetic sunscreens can prove irritating for those with sensitive skin. As India Knight, skin care guru for the *Sunday Times*, wrote, "A chemical sunscreen gets absorbed into your body; a mineral sunscreen sits on top of skin bouncing rays off, but washes off." High-factor mineral screens used to be thick and chalky white, but more recent launches are sheer and much less noticeable. During the course of my interviews and reading, a preference for factor 50 sunscreens for babies and children seems to be the go-to solution for people with lupus.

Dental Problems

Mouth ulcers are a hallmark of lupus, as discussed, but even with excellent oral hygiene, higher levels of gum problems and dental decay can also be part of the mouth problems associated with lupus. A US blog, where a systemic lupus sufferer thanked her rheumatologist and her dentist for their care and help, was my first indication that teeth were susceptible to damage by lupus. The first signs of such problems for me came when a back molar crumbled away one evening some months after the onset of my serious flare, and regular dental work has been necessary ever since. My dentist also understands that with constant pain elsewhere, that extra pain relief for dental work is helpful.

A contributory factor to dental damage can be the leaching of calcium caused by corticosteroids. Corticosteroids increase calcium excretion by the kidneys and decrease the absorption of calcium through the stomach. As previously mentioned, in order to protect bone density and ultimately increased risk of bone breakage for those on corticosteroids for more than a few weeks, along with dental health, it is important to take calcium and vitamin D supplements supported by a nutrient-rich diet (please see further detail in chapter 11, "Optimum Nutrition for Lupus").

A lack of saliva associated with Sjögren's syndrome can also increase acid in the mouth, further promoting cavities. It is therefore advisable to schedule regular trips to a trusted dentist to protect your teeth if you have systemic lupus erythematosus, and you may need extra oral hygiene products such as high-fluoride toothpaste and even three-monthly topical fluoride treatments to prevent cavities.

Fertility and Pregnancy Complications

For women of childbearing age, lupus can cause miscarriages and birth complications. The autoimmune element whereby the body attacks its own healthy cells unfortunately includes fetuses in the womb. "There is an increased risk of [fetal] loss and miscarriages in lupus patients" (Lupus UK 2015). Although more than half of all lupus pregnancies will be without complications, in the UK, all lupus pregnancies are now routinely considered high risk. One of the most critical reasons for raising the profile of lupus is that, in my own experience, it is not a test automatically carried out in cases of multiple miscarriage, even though by some estimates, one out of five lupus pregnancies results in miscarriage.

In addition, a common feature of lupus is disrupted periods, and during some flares, they can halt altogether. Evidence also suggests a worsening of lupus symptoms prior to the normal date of your period, as you might experience premenstrual symptoms. Even if your periods have halted, there may still be a pattern of aggravated symptoms around the date that your period used to occur.

There has also been some research carried out into what appears to be a higher rate of false-positive smear tests in systemic lupus erythematosus patients, perhaps because the inflammation associated with lupus may influence the cells around the cervix. A study reporting in January 2015 found that 12.5 percent of SLE patients had abnormal smears versus none in the control group (Al Sherbeni 2015). However, the study also pointed out that lupus patients had a higher rate of all types of cancer overall than non-lupus patients, with the rate of malignancy notably higher in the first five years post-diagnosis than for those who had lupus for more than ten years. However, it is not clear whether this is down to the condition or the medications associated with the condition, which included immunosuppressants in some of the patients examined.

The study concluded that regular smear tests, especially in the first five years after diagnosis, were advisable. In addition, the statistics are further muddled by the variability with which patients are diagnosed with lupus, making the five-year window something of a movable target. The conclusion is perhaps simpler, which is to be aware of the higher incidence of false-positive smear tests when reacting to the news of an anomalous result, and to have the confidence to ask for a second opinion or further checks on the health of the cervix and the womb before jumping to negative conclusions.

While this examination of the secondary symptoms of lupus is not exhaustive and is not intended to be a replacement for expert medical commentary, it does set out to answer as many of the leading queries that I have found from my own journey, from my interviews, and across the Internet. Please find below a summary list of other possible physical symptoms that can occur with systemic lupus erythematosus and discoid lupus erythematosus with systemic complications, outside of the official diagnostic list:

- Pain
- Fatigue

- Nausea
- Feverishness
- Lupus fog
- Esophageal complications
- Hair loss
- Susceptibility to circadian rhythms and barometric pressure
- Skin sensitivity
- Dental problems
- Fertility, pregnancy, and gynecological problems

It is my hope that this first part, "Understanding Lupus," informs, clarifies, and reduces your sense of initial confusion as you or someone you love or care for faces this often-complicated disease. Perhaps it has given guidance that you may have missed or at least reassurance that you are not alone in what you are experiencing. The ramifications of lupus can sometimes leave patients bewildered and overwhelmed. Together with experiencing this firsthand, I have seen it repeatedly in the blogs, the message boards, the forums, and heard it from fellow lupus patients. These fundamental facts aim to make the often unfamiliar and unknown known.

I gradually cancelled my external life. Fortunately, I had recently completed one role working with severely disabled young people, but I had started looking for another. A post-qualifying part-time psychotherapy course booked for the summer was thankfully delayed until the autumn so my deposit was returned and my work for two leading UK mental health charities was forced on hold. There was also no option but to resign the chair of a local voluntary organization and shelve plans to return to help a mental health user development facility in the next county. My hobbies, which included walking my dogs for miles in all weather, were now nearly all impossible.

My daily world had shrunk to the sofa and a small side table next to it, which carried my essentials within easy reach, namely a glass of water, the TV remote, and some lip balm, along with a small handmade ceramic dog curled asleep, which was made by a local artist and given to me by my nearest neighbor as a get-well present. Neighbors, friends, and family would phone, and I would take the call if I could. We would visit for short spells so as not to tire me out, drawing up an armchair and telling me about life outside. Through them and the television, I lived vicariously.

As the weeks advanced and summer approached, it became clear, given the level of ongoing pain, that the dose of corticosteroids was too low. So my London consultant proposed doubling the amount of stomach liner omeprazole to enable a higher dose of prednisolone. Unfortunately, two weeks into the new regime, I woke to find myself covered head to foot, literally from the tips of my ears to my toes, in an itchy red rash. London suggested that I get immediately to my local general practice to get a diagnosis.

The rash looked so spectacular that the doctor called in a second opinion and then a third in the form of the head of the practice, giving rise to the situation where I found myself seated, partially undressed in a camisole, with three doctors standing in a semicircle around me, all staring. They concluded it was a severe allergic reaction to the increase in the stomach liner; told me to stop taking the omeprazole immediately; and prescribed a new stomach liner, ranitidine hydrochloride, often marketed under the brand name Zantac, plus topical corticosteroid cream. Their prescription worked, and the rash stopped in its tracks, but it still took over three months for it to disappear completely, and this highlights the potential sensitivity of the lupus system and lupus skin.

Because I was remaining in chronic and continuous pain, desperately weak, fatigued and needing care, it was concluded that the twenty-five milligrams of corticosteroids per day were not working, so my London-based consultant recommended that I take the new lupus drug mycophenolate mofetil. This, as I have mentioned, is a new-wave medicine for lupus, previously an immunosuppressant drug and originally used to prevent rejection of kidneys, livers, and hearts in organ transplants.

Three days into taking mycophenolate, the fog cleared, the pain subsided, and wonderfully my energy rebounded. Delighted, I felt cured and could see regaining my strength and being able to return to my old life. I remember standing in the kitchen, elated that a solution to my desperate situation had finally been found. The nightmare would soon be over …

Unfortunately, my euphoria was short-lived, as I started vomiting eleven days later. My general practitioner instructed me to stop taking the drug, and under direction from London, I then left a gap of some three months before trying it again in oral solution. Heartbreakingly, the same outcome took place; I felt great for ten days, but after eleven days, my body could no longer tolerate it. With massive regret, the new drug had to be abandoned. Subsequent research has revealed that other lupus patients can have difficulty tolerating mycophenolate mofetil, including adverse impacts on white blood cell counts after over a year.

Hugely disappointed, we went to London for a consultation and were told that my flare rated in the top two percent of flares that lupus patients could experience and that in the spring, I had been "fading fast" toward death. We were also told also that I had failed to be able to tolerate the only leading-edge drug available. We were advised that therefore the route to recovery from my severe flare could be more arduous because the alternative to mycophenolate was an older and less efficient immunosuppressant called azathioprine, which was a retired chemotherapy drug for cancer. Azathioprine accrues in the system gradually and therefore takes a lot longer to show its benefits. Indeed, in conclusion, my London consultant told my husband and me, "You need to consider that this might be as good as it gets and that you may never recover much further from here."

Being told that I needed to accept the reality of how ill I had been and to appreciate being alive is perhaps understandable, but it did not advance me much from my severely disabled state. Driving away from that appointment, the realization hit me that somehow I needed to find a different way to recover, but desperately weak, bundled up in rugs and pillows and dosed up, I had no idea how. Nevertheless, something needed to change soon; otherwise, I could imagine my incredibly supportive and protective husband having a frank conversation with my consultant.

While I am sure that the consultant was hugely successful with many other patients—indeed, support staff told me so—recent meetings had not started well for us. It seemed that he could not remember the details of my case, nor had he read my notes before the meetings, perhaps because he was always late and rushed. So he needed reminding of the salient facts of my situation and this in the context of our having driven over one and a half hours and through London traffic to reach him. Having worked in a professional capacity, knowing that the other party is not fully briefed is a factor that you get to recognize, and to encounter this when your life literally depends upon the meeting is distressing. You just feel so powerless. Complex drug therapy is not my subject, and at the time, I had not educated myself to lupus medicines and their background, so I felt our position to be invidious.

Perhaps my circumstances were particularly difficult in that I seemed especially sensitive, but it is my profound belief that being told that your situation is stagnant at best, irretrievable at worst, is no help at all. In fact, it is damaging to your mental state and to the morale of those who care for you and love you.

As we drove down the embankment, with the majestic River Thames on my left, toward Parliament Square and Big Ben, I knew that change had become urgent.

PART II

A Mental and Emotional Journey

CHAPTER 5

The Impact of Pain on the Brain

Illness is not something a person has. It's another way of being.
—Jonathan Miller

The physical facts are only the foundation of a thorough exploration of lupus, and this second part turns the spotlight on its mental and emotional implications, which are often profound. Initially, it is valuable to examine the impact of long-term pain on the brain. Acute pain is defined as essentially temporary, such as when you receive an injury to a part of the body, as with severe bruising, pulling a muscle, spraining tendons, breaking bones, or cutting or burning the skin. Chronic pain is different because it stays and is defined as persistent pain lasting longer than twelve weeks.

Statistics show that approximately 1.5 billion people worldwide live with lasting pain. The American Chronic Pain Association estimated that 100 million Americans endure this type of pain or, to put it another way, one in ten have experienced pain every day for three months or more. It is an epidemic, and recently the *British Medical Journal* quoted a systematic review that concluded that approximately 28 million adults in the UK suffer from chronic pain, or over a third of the population (Fayaz 2016). Recently, in 2017, the American Academy of Pain Medicine stated that more Americans suffer from chronic pain than diabetes, heart disease, and cancer combined.

Since the early 1990s, there have been huge strides made into research as to how the brain works, led by advances in functional magnetic resonance imaging (fMRI). fMRI is a specialized form of brain and body scan, and researchers and clinicians have been able to study the processes of the brain noninvasively for the first time because fMRI does not require sedation, the injection of highlighting fluids, or exposure to radiation. This new research technique was built on the existing MRI technology and on discoveries as to the properties of oxygen-rich blood.

Deoxygenated blood is more magnetic than oxygenated blood, and the difference in the signals can therefore be calibrated. Then researchers discovered that when neurons are activated in a particular part of the brain, blood flow surges into that area as oxygen-rich blood and pushes out oxygen-depleted blood. Researchers can now identify when an area of the brain is active or in use because blood flow (or the hemodynamic response) to that area also increases. Then using color coding, scans can map what areas of the brain are influenced by a particular stimulus. This is meaningful to this book because fMRI has been able to track which parts of the brain are impacted not only by pain but also by relaxation techniques and even meditation.

In 2008, Dante Chialvo, the associate research professor of physiology at the Feinberg School at Northwestern University in the United States, and his team found that in healthy people, the key areas of the brain all work together in harmony. When one region is active, the other regions go quiet, but in the brains of people with chronic pain, the frontal region of the brain, that which is primarily associated with emotion, never quietens down.

Chialvo therefore noted, "If you are a chronic pain patient, you have pain twenty-four hours a day, seven days a week, every minute of your life." This was my reality. My pain could be well controlled, fairly controlled, or not controlled, and there were frequent spikes when, despite all my efforts, it spiraled completely out of control, creating pain and nausea crises, which then left me utterly depleted for several days. Pain felt like the most difficult authority figure I had ever encountered, one that had to be pandered to, cajoled, and second-guessed, but often to no avail. As Stephen King remarked in *Duma Key,* "There is no tyrant as merciless as pain."

When my sister-in-law Angela came to stay from Australia, she read the paper in the armchair next to me, keeping me company with deep kindness as I dozed on the sofa, having taken pain relief. Yes, still on that sofa, propped up with pillows and covered in a fluffy rug. When I woke up, she reported that I was moaning and talking about the pain even as I slept. Chialvo's research showed that this nonstop pain shows up in the frontal cortex as a failure to shut down … ever. He identified that this continuous processing not only wears out the neurons in this area of the cortex but that it also alters the harmonious functioning of the brain as a whole (Chialvo 2008). Furthermore, he went on to hypothesize that this disharmony can lead to problems such as depression, anxiety, and insomnia in patients suffering from lasting pain.

Support for this idea that chronic pain actually damages the functionality of the brain was reinforced by research on mice, published in 2012, which showed that pain harms the hippocampus, the region of the brain responsible for learning, memory, and processing the emotions, disrupting its ability to produce new neurons. This links to reports from people in pain experiencing disordered thinking, poorer concentration, and memory loss. I called it my "scrambled egg brain," something totally at variance with the reliable machine that had organized my previous busy, highly productive life, in which I had passed my most recent academic qualifications with distinction.

In 2017, *New Scientist* reported on a new study, again on mice, using the latest neuroimaging techniques, which showed that chronic pain induced changes in the regions of their brains linked to depression and anxiety. The mice "became hypersensitive to harmless touch" and then "developed anxiety and depression-like behaviors" (Ananthaswamy 2017). While recognizing that the link to anxiety and depression may not hold in human cases and that further research into the human implications is therefore required (and I feel sorry for the mice), the research is acknowledged to be another step forward in the understanding of how continuous pain may disrupt brain function.

The finding of hypersensitivity to harmless touch strikes a chord with me, given my intolerance for anything that would add to my discomfort to any degree because of the proximity to the pain threshold. Because I could not bear any tightness or restrictions from clothing or the feel of seams, labels, or zips, I wore a series of loose pajama-like outfits. Too weak to source or try things on for myself, Angela went shopping for me in Melbourne and mailed casual separates to me from Australia, while my mother provided the softest wraps and shawls.

In his study of 1,006 patients in chronic pain, Alejandro Salazar noted that he and his team "observed a high prevalence of undiagnosed mood disorders in chronic musculoskeletal pain patients" (Salazar 2013). Indeed, he put the figure at about 75 percent, and you should bear in mind that with lupus, pain may be one of the two most common symptoms along with fatigue but there are other quality-of-life reducing factors. "Chronic pain affects every aspect of an individual's life, including their relationships with others, employment, and ability to participate in everyday activities. Clearly, when any condition has this level of impact on our patient's lives and on those of their loved ones, it's no wonder they are likely to experience negative emotions" (Moyle 2016).

So the potential mental ramifications for lupus patients can be huge. Make no mistake: this chronic illness can be a psychological boot camp, an assault course for the emotions, where there is no quarter given and nowhere to hide.

Wendy's Story

"It is very hard to pin it down to one emotion. Frustration: at not being the strong (physically and emotionally) person I was before and frustration with the fatigue and total lethargy every day. I want more energy. I want to do more. Sadness: that life will never be the same again. Grief: at that loss of the old me, the real me. Determination: to do my best for my husband and my children and, of course, myself. Guilt: for my family, that I cannot do more or be better for them. Fear: of what the future might hold. It's different emotions every day. Sometimes you can deal with them, and sometimes, when you are already low and struggling, they can totally overwhelm you."

My psychotherapeutic training and experience gave me heightened awareness of the changes in my mental state, but it did not remove these unfamiliar emotions or reduce their intensity. Firstly, this examination of the range of feelings that can be triggered by lupus looks first and foremost to verify and validate your own possible reactions; secondly, to let you see that you are not alone in feeling as you do; and thirdly, and importantly, to give you the permission to say, "See, it's not me. It's my illness!"

"The real me," as Wendy so brilliantly identifies it, is still in there—just battered by relentless symptoms.

Denial and Stoicism

> Even as your body betrays you, your mind denies it.
> —Sara Gruen, *Water for Elephants*

Hiding is an instinctive initial reaction that can take the form of denial. Given my British predilection for understatement, denial for me is assuming that everyone around me is probably overreacting. When my liver specialist reassured me triumphantly that the latest batch of tests proved that I did not need a liver transplant, my immediate reaction was, "Of course I wasn't going to need a liver transplant! Don't be silly. I could have told you that."

I didn't actually voice this, but I could tell that my consultant was deflated by my lack of relief at this potentially life-changing news. In retrospect, I see a self-protection mechanism at work.

As a coping technique, denial is understandable, harmless even, but overt stoicism can take an emotional toll on both you and those around you. Maintaining quiet fortitude in all circumstances when facing this illness can prove counterproductive. Saying that you are fine when you are not and trying to spin things for the benefit of others is often a waste of energy. Those around you are usually not fooled. Calm clarification is not the same as self-indulgence, and your loved ones, family, and friends will appreciate your honesty. It will also save them having to second-guess how you are feeling. Silence can build a wall up against those trying to understand and help.

In addition, as this can be a life-threatening condition, if denial is preventing you from seeking and pursuing treatment, then it is potentially dangerous. When seeking diagnosis and treatment, you should have faith that you are a strong and capable person and that something is just not right with your body. Fundamentally, trust that your instincts are correct.

Unfortunately, as we have already illustrated, many with lupus have to fight to get their symptoms recognized and diagnosed, and sometimes they have to continue that battle to get ongoing treatment with compassion and full understanding. Disbelief from the start can set a precedent and put those with lupus psychologically on the back foot from the outset. Also, any tendency to "people please," which is not an unusual default position, can further complicate matters.

"Keeping a stiff upper lip" is traditionally described as a British attribute, and it is a reference to the tendency for the lower lip to quiver involuntarily in times of extreme nervousness. I watched a lead witness in a courtroom, under cross-examination by the barrister, hold his hand underneath his chin because his bottom lip trembled so much. His uncertainty was justified as his past actions were revealed under questioning, and he went on to lose the case. A stiff upper lip is therefore the opposite and, traditionally, implies strength and huge self-restraint when faced with a difficult situation.

Cultural norms celebrate overt self-reliance and stoicism in the face of adversity. Many with lupus have faced judgment that they should be mentally stronger and show more grit throughout their lives, when in fact they have been struggling against a profound hidden disability for years, making it through without the health that the majority take for granted. During the course of my research, lupus patients have imparted phrases that they have encountered, such as "being self-indulgent," "overexaggerating," "attention seeking," and, perhaps the most startling, "throwing a pity party."

It is a situation exacerbated by the fact that without the distinctive malar rash, which as we know is not always present and often transitory, those with lupus can often look normal and show no physical evidence of the internal ravages of their disease. It is one of a category of medical conditions that is often referred to as "invisible illnesses." The problem with the lack of physical evidence can lead to negative judgments by those ignorant of the true implications. Then, as Kaleidoscope Fighting Lupus identifies, "The invisible illness sufferer is often labelled lazy while disease wreaks havoc inside their body."

These factors add up to mean that contrary to being weaker and less determined than average, those with lupus have often been, in practice and out of necessity, stronger and more resilient than the norm. From interviewing, researching, and participating in the field, it is actually clear that patients are often understating their mental strength in the face of cruel symptoms. I feel privileged to have witnessed stories of great courage and resilience. Not only are patients unaware of this, but to compound matters, they usually also feel terribly responsible for all the things they feel that they *should* be achieving.

Shame and Guilt

Pain has a way of clipping our wings and keeping us from being able to fly.
—William P. Young, *The Shack*

In 2015, Julie Turner-Cobb studied the emotions of patients with chronic pain versus a control group and found "significantly greater levels of shame, guilt, fear of negative evaluation, and mental defeat … compared to controls" (Turner-Cobb 2015).

The sudden sense of powerlessness can be devastating. Far from coping, resourceful, tenacious, optimistic me felt regularly out of options, with my emotional equilibrium shaken and my resilient core under sustained attack. As the days became weeks, there was no option but to crawl back to the sofa, pull up a rug, and allow the body to rebuild at its own glacial pace. The realization had to be that sometimes it is okay simply to survive. As William Hague wrote in his biography of British Prime Minister Pitt the Younger, "Celebrate your ability to weather the storm."

However, it was very hard to be positive at the start. Obsessively retracing my steps, I felt stupid to have broken myself, feeling such an idiot to have pushed myself so far and hard that I had crashed my body somehow. My mind replayed what could possibly have gone awry, what warnings signs had been missed that would have pulled me back from the brink before tumbling down so far. In ignorance of the basic facts of the disease at that time, I had instead an overwhelming sense of having done something wrong, thereby adding guilt to my roster of misery.

I had also lost the status of a job in any form, especially that of a good homemaker, which I prized highly, and could see no prospect of being able to work at anything meaningful ever again in my broken state.

In American culture, independence and self-reliance are rightly celebrated, as embodied in Ralph Waldo Emerson's famous phrase "Hitch your wagon to a star" ("American Civilization," *The Atlantic* 1862), which encapsulates the freedom and determination of the pioneering spirit. In direct contrast, severe illness traps you in your own body and you find yourself reliant on others at every turn. It is easy to feel helpless and hopeless, particularly as the days extend to weeks and then months and your body responds at its own snail's pace. Unable to do maybe even the simplest tasks, you are forced to sit and watch while others do it around you. You feel frustrated that you are unable to recover quickly. You have gone from someone who looks after others—relied on by them to achieve goals and to forge forward in life—to feeling like a burden.

In modern times, continuous self-improvement is the norm, and the media, particularly the social media phenomenon, can make competitive comparison a daily event. As we know, the majority of lupus sufferers are women, and they expect to achieve much on many levels, optimizing their appearances, careers, relationships, and homes. We are in fact all multitaskers and high achievers but often completely dismissive of these daily and weekly successes. We take it all for granted and then, on top of that, presume constant improvement. We totally dismiss our independent lives in which we jump in and out of cars and on and off trains, meet deadlines, keep commitments, and shoulder enormous responsibilities. Suddenly, it had all come to a juddering halt for me, and I found myself unable to put on my own socks!

Despair

In a real dark night of the soul, it is always three o'clock in the morning.
—F. Scott Fitzgerald, *The Crack Up*

In the face of relentless pain and fatigue, my natural sense of optimism and resilience were sucked out of me. This enemy felt bigger than I was. Due to the exhaustion, more than anything, you begin to distance yourself as a protection mechanism because you simply don't have the energy to worry anymore. I started to emotionally detach from my loved ones as I got weaker and weaker. Looking back, I empathize with P. J. O'Rourke's words "I looked death in the face. All right, I didn't. I glimpsed him in a crowd."

The nights were especially difficult because I had developed a particular pattern of abruptly waking up out of a drugged deep sleep at around three o'clock. Intense anxiety would press heavy on my chest, and it was then, in those dark early hours of the morning, that suicidal thoughts came unbidden and gained a terrifying logic all of their own. I had a sense of looking back at the world from inside a long dark tunnel, and hour by difficult hour, day by difficult day, I moved further and further down. At my most vulnerable, the feelings of uselessness and being a burden gave rise to a warped logic that it would be much more efficient if I did just die. Never in my life previously had I been suicidal, but my counselling training recognized immediately the seriousness of these new thoughts, even though I felt powerless to prevent them.

However, at the foot of my bed stood my husband, and it began to occur to me that he seemed to mind awfully that I was so unwell and imperative to him that I simply existed, terrible encumbrance or not. The look of concern on his face was so intense that it reached through the fog surrounding me, running counter to my logic of peaceful capitulation, shining like a beacon at the far mouth of the tunnel, lighting my way back.

My dog kept faithful guard at my feet like a small sphinx, and sometimes the terrier, tired of hunting, would join us in his bed on the floor and they would both snore gently. As the days progressed, the realization grew that even if broken and useless, my husband seemed to want me, and even if I could not feed or walk them, the dogs also seemed blissfully happy in my company. So the roles of wife and dog companion were there, if only hanging by a thread.

Depression

> These are the times that try men's souls.
> —Thomas Paine, *The Crisis*

"Depression is frequently undiagnosed ... particularly in patients suffering from chronic pain" (Salazar 2013), and he and his team go on to say that pain and depression often coexist in an estimated 30 percent to 60 percent of lupus cases.

A sense of high anxiety or doom is a clinical symptom of certain life-threatening conditions, including heart attacks and snakebites, and from my experience and research, I believe that low mood and depression are also clear psychological symptoms of lupus flares. Lupus appears to cloak lives in negative feelings, and these intensify during bouts of disease activity.

Many patients have reported deep and sudden negative feelings such as extreme sadness, tearfulness, suicidal ideation, intense anxiety, and despair, completely at variance with their normally optimistic, resilient characters.

This book contains stories from ex- military officers, nurses, financiers, marketing executives, and craftsmen, to name but a few, who have led dynamic, highly resourceful lives before being overcome with lupus flares. Given my training, I could self-diagnose depression but initially could not see any solutions. The latest research in 2017 concluded, "Systemic lupus erythematosus patients are at high risk for depression and anxiety" (Zang 2017).

Given that severe lupus can disrupt the whole fabric of your life, from employment prospects to hobbies and socializing, it is not surprising that it gives rise to two key traits of clinical depression, namely feelings of helplessness and hopelessness. What also must be added into the mix is the fact that corticosteroids such as prednisolone at doses in excess of twenty milligrams or more can have depression as a possible side effect. In those early weeks and months, having been catapulted from an incredibly fulfilling and active midlife into the world of a frail ninety-year-old, I could see no way forward.

CHAPTER 6

Erratic Progress

Believe in miracle and cures and healing wells.
—Seamus Heaney, *The Cure at Troy*

Three weeks after the devastating consultation in London and the demise of hope given my intolerance for mycophenolate, I received a call from the head of my local general practice, asking me to come in and see him. An arrangement had previously been made that my London consultant would keep them informed of my treatment and that they might help with sourcing a local neurologist to assess small numb patches on my right hand and right foot. My local general practice and the associated emergency doctors and nurses had been unfailingly helpful when it came to supporting my pain and nausea.

Apart from his belief that he could recommend an excellent neurologist, my general practitioner had been thoroughly confused by the letter he had received from London because he found it full of errors about my medications and their dosages. This letter added to our concerns about the level of care being provided by London, and armed with the referral to a neurologist, we tried to edge our way ahead.

The neurologist came across as kind and thorough and, having completed my examination, wanted to work in tandem with my lupus specialist. Put on the spot and against the backdrop of our recent concerns, we found ourselves being open about the problems we were encountering.

It emerged from the conversation that the neurologist was used to working closely with a local rheumatologist. It was pointed out that this would avoid my having to go to London, a moot point because to get the right care, I would have travelled gladly, but journeying in discomfort to disappointment was just adding insult to injury. After further consideration, we decided to go ahead and seek a second opinion.

With my husband with me to help explain my case, we went to see the new local rheumatologist. In direct comparison to my recent London consultations, she had read everything sent through beforehand, taken extensive notes, and examined the detail of my medications. We agreed on a new system that layered in new safeguards for the range of lupus symptoms, so a daily aspirin and hydroxychloroquine were added. For some unaccountable reason, given what I now understand to be its baseline benefits and its long-term ability to prevent organ damage, hydroxychloroquine was missing from my prescriptions. As my muscles began to seize in the hard chair, she concluded that I needed a high dose of intravenous corticosteroids almost immediately due to my poor state. She assessed an emergency that had to be remedied within the week. In great contrast, her whole approach appeared thorough and dynamic, but above all, she gave me a glimpse of optimism:

"Do you think I can improve, then?" Asked tentatively.

"Of course you will!" Said with her shoulders back and with confidence.

"Oh, I thought that was me done, so to speak." Said quietly.

Glancing up, she gave a robust smile, and my heart lifted. We had been gifted our first positive news in a while and were seeing the first ray of hope.

Due to the range of symptoms, from mild to severe and from aches and pains to organ failure, every experience of lupus is unique. Due to all the variables, each case manifests in a highly personal way, which also means that no two healing journeys are likely to be the same. This is primarily a physical journey, but one with profound mental and emotional implications. Therefore, a positive support structure is essential. The situation is even more critical if you find yourself advised by someone you feel is not on top of your case and seemingly unable, or unwilling, to understand the depth of your physical predicament.

You need people around you who believe in your potential to improve, and it is not for any advisor to rule out personal resilience. Your confidence in the team looking after you is fundamental. You need to have faith in them, and they need to have faith in you. Trust your instincts about your care. Molly's Fund Fighting Lupus states, "We encourage you to be your strongest advocate," and looking back, I now appreciate that when you hit a wall, it may be time to seek an alternative.

Two days later, I spent several hours in my local hospital connected to a drip being pumped with an emergency dose of intravenous corticosteroids. Returning home into the arms of my family and friends, I suffered no negative side effects and waited for the benefits of the new regime to filter through my system.

The first benefit of the intravenous treatment saw the lupus fog lift and my interest in the world around me intensify. My hands had been so clawed, particularly the right one, that it proved difficult for me to hold on to things. My arms could take little weight and would quickly become painful holding up a newspaper or a book for any length of time. I acquired a small tablet that came in a case that I could prop over slightly bent knees, removing the weight from my hands and allowing my legs to remain in their comfortable position raised on the sofa or bed.

Although hardly able to write, and then only shakily and with great effort, tapping and swiping on the tablet came easy, and it could be picked up and put down depending on how I felt. A little window on the whole world now opened up, satisfying my hunger for information; it also gave me the ability to start researching lupus. With some more energy also at my disposal, I could now shop online, researching purchases with new care and diligence, having previously, prior to my illness, been so pressed for time. Starting to reconnect with family and friends via email and social media, I began to build a circle that would send me news and pictures about their lives. I saw pictures of major construction projects, tables set for beautiful dinner parties, outfits for balls; I traveled the globe secondhand. I am incredibly grateful that I have been seriously ill in the age of the Internet and small mobile devices.

My dog had previously curled herself up on the opposite end of the sofa during the day, close but not impeding me, as being constricted in any way by a heavy dog would have been painful. A few days after the infusion, she sometimes started to move closer, pressing against my legs and putting a soft head within distance of a hand for a stroke. She seemed to know that I was now strong enough, and I took this as a sign of progress and felt encouraged.

The discoid rashes at the base of my neck faded, although they would flare up at odd intervals. My swallowing improved, but I remained vigilant to prevent choking. My appetite was erratic and frequently disrupted by pain and exhaustion. Crises of pain and nausea were regular. My joints would swell on a whim, and standing for any time was still beyond me. My body lagged far behind my brain and my desire to get better, but the sense of total hopelessness retreated. Overall, I was less overwhelmed and more alert, despite the one constant: pain.

Uncertainty

Some leading lupus websites encourage patients to keep a diary to track possible instigators of increased disease activity, which include the following:

- Exposure to sunlight and UVB overhead lighting
- Food allergies or reactions (see part III)
- Overdoing it/lifting something heavy/twisting
- Overintense therapy
- Shortage of or disrupted sleep
- Airborne allergen
- Menstrual cycle

Diligently I tracked all of the possibilities, especially dietary reactions, given that I had been officially diagnosed as allergic to gluten. In reality, I could feel worse with no apparent cause and have good days and bad days without rhyme or reason. I could find few patterns to get a handle on. My husband is an experimental physicist by education, but he could detect no consistent trends either. The hardest part can be the not knowing how you are going to feel when you open your eyes on any given morning, a point corroborated by Nadia who wrote to me, "The most common emotion that I feel is uncertainty—not knowing how I will feel from one day to the next."

At worst, I would awake in severe pain, triggering nausea. Then it would be a scramble to get the sickness under control as a first port of call. This meant that nothing could be planned to a specific timeframe and that all appointments had to be made with caveats and the ability to cancel. I could not even leave messages on answering machines in case the pain had taken over by the time they called back.

Frustration

There is a built-in expectation that you will get better, day by day or at least week by week, but the reality of lupus is far more chaotic. Many factors can influence improvement, and there is a sense of playing a giant game where forward momentum is made for a few days or even a week to ten days, only to fall back on a turn of the dice, suddenly in crisis, utterly demoralized.

At times, the process reminded me of the Greek legend of Sisyphus, an ancient Greek king of what is modern-day Corinth. His violent and avaricious behavior upset the Greek gods, and as punishment, he was forced to roll a huge boulder up a hill in the underworld, only to have it roll back down again, when close to the top, for all eternity. This sense of utter frustration and of never making any real improvement seemed to typify my day-to-day experience of living with lupus. Good progress felt like two steps forward, one back.

It became clear when I reached out to the Lupus UK forum that I was not alone in experiencing acute frustration. Leesy represented many on the Lupus UK forum when she wrote, "Frustration is my most common emotion because you feel like you can do things you did before, then you feel completely exhausted when you do them!"

Research has identified a tendency for those with chronic pain to demonstrate "impatience with pain—and belief that an individual should be doing better than they are" (McAllister 2015). With my brain so much more alert, I had to come to terms with the fact that my body could not be controlled at will and I needed to find a way to move forward, accommodating its unreliability. I needed to accept that mini-flares were part of an overall recovery from a major flare, and indeed of the condition itself.

Isolation

Your world can get smaller because you spend a great deal of time confined to your home. You can start to feel trapped. No longer able to go out to work every day or to socialize regularly, many begin to feel isolated. Imom wrote to me: "I am just sad that I am not the person I was just several years ago, and I also feel isolation because I cannot repay dinner parties or host parties in turn. Also, I can't keep up with them on shopping outings."

Many feel embarrassed at having to explain their symptoms, and their confidence is eroded by having to make repeated excuses. This can therefore intensify feelings of loneliness.

The Dollhouse Reaction

Your world can become centered on the few rooms that you occupy most. Over time, life becomes miniaturized, and I call this "the dollhouse reaction." This can lead to mildly obsessive feelings about your immediate environment, which, if you were busy, you would not notice and certainly would not prioritize. You can become preoccupied with small details. For example, I had some light switches that were pressure activated in one room only, but with my compromised hand and often stumbling around in pain, I found them very difficult to use, especially at night. In the end, I had to get them changed to the same easy system as elsewhere.

Similarly, unable to bend down and get a dustpan and brush or a vacuum cleaner to pick up dust or debris on the floor, their presence would annoy me intensely. While these may seem minor points, the obsessive-compulsive disorder (OCD) mind-set is not a healthy one, and as such, it is an extension of the helplessness that underpins damaging feelings of isolation and depression.

Agoraphobia

An extension of the dollhouse reaction can become a sense of anxiety when you do leave the house. Initially, my nascent agoraphobia manifested in a sense of mild panic that I had forgotten something or left something on in the house that could cause a fire. I began to appreciate that my panicky feelings would kick in about five minutes after leaving the house when being driven down the road. I identified that the overall situation was not helped by the fact that I once asked my husband, "Why is it that every time I leave the house, someone sticks a needle in me?"

The reality of being severely ill can be a seemingly never-ending round of medical appointments, tests, and essential treatments rather than going out to do anything pleasant and rewarding.

Panic Attacks

You may become aware that you are making excuses to avoid going out, beyond being trapped by pain, fatigue, and weakness. Reluctance and avoidance are manageable, but if you find it impossible to leave the house at all, then this is a warning sign, as are signs of a panic attack on leaving the house or while out. Feelings of dependency and fragility can erode confidence and leave some feeling very uncertain. I have corresponded with sufferers who are often overwhelmed with anxiety, despite being confident and outgoing people prior to the onset of their acute lupus symptoms.

Symptoms of panic attacks are as follows:

- Intense feeling of anxiety and stress
- Rapid breathing escalating to hyperventilation, which is breathlessness, through to a sense of having difficulty breathing
- A rapid heartbeat
- Feeling hot and sweating
- Feeling nauseated or actually being sick

If symptoms escalate to these levels, then you are advised to seek professional help either from your doctor or from a counsellor or psychotherapist so that they can make a further assessment.

Fear of Missing Out, or FOMO

In the same category is a mental anxiety state called FOMO, or fear of missing out, a term officially added to the *Oxford English Dictionary* in 2013. It is a clever acronym "coined to describe that anxious feeling that can arise when you feel that there is a more exciting prospect that is happening elsewhere, and unfortunately you are not there," according to Aarti Gupta, PsyD, who is a clinical director at the Center for Anxiety Disorders in Los Altos, California. While Dr. Gupta's focus is the modern obsession with social media, the chronically ill experience a similar sensation because, as she points out, the situation taps in to our basic survival instincts—back to a time when knowing what the tribe was doing or being separated from your group could prove critical to existence. We all therefore have a deep inbuilt anxiety about being left out, left behind, or abandoned.

Dr. Gupta suggests that recognizing the problem and its source is a good starting point. Making the subconscious conscious is the jump-off for any therapy. She then recommends practicing mindfulness, which we discuss in more detail later, as helpful. Establishing a new communication network that accommodates your illness is also beneficial.

Developing a hobby or interest in something current can make you feel more connected, and you can join discussion groups, online forums, or healing groups. You may need to explore fresh ways to share news and information easily when you are physically able. With kind flexibility, my good friends and neighbors understood that if they phoned and the answering machine clicked in, it was best to leave a message. This would either allow me the time to get to the phone, as I moved very slowly, or to get back to them when feeling better. Emails worked well, with family and friends sending me updates from around the world about what they were doing, as I have already mentioned. Certain friends were also wonderful at sending humorous videos or pictures to make me laugh and were wise to my love of animals, plants, and flowers. By degrees, I built a rich new platform of interaction that substantially reduced my feelings of missing out.

Being in pain does not mean that you should give up on love, light, and laughter. On the contrary, you need these gifts more than ever! You need to find systems to rebuild your confidence in yourself, in what life has to offer, and find fresh ways to feel positive when you wake. In the case of the severely disabled students that I felt privileged to counsel on placement, the counselling team and the staff of the college always avoided the negative and focused instead on what the students *could* do, rather than their limitations. It seemed clear to me that severe pain and chronic illness needed the same constructive approach.

At this point, I could count on an incredible close personal support structure and an excellent and trusted medical team, consisting of an uplifting new local rheumatologist, my unfailing general practice team, and wise community nurses. My training as a counsellor and psychotherapist also gave me some extra resources. However, my situation still felt dire and I remained desperate for mental solace as well as physical progress. Therefore, some eighteen months after the onset of my huge flare, I set out to find brand-new systems and methods to allow me to cope better.

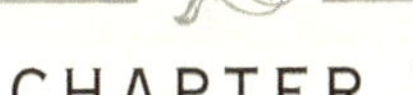

CHAPTER 7

Psychological Interventions

The integration of psychological interventions with
the treatment of chronic pain is essential.
—Dr Allen Lebovits, PhD

Part I of this book sets out to explain the physical implications of this condition and the medical treatment for it, while the beginning of part II looks to validate the knock-on emotional and psychological challenges that it presents. Both seek to provide you with clarity about what you may face. Analysis of the possible mental repercussions shows that you have every right to feel negative, battered by symptoms and circumstance, but from this point on, there is a pressing requirement for reassurance that there are ways forward. There is a need to show that despite everything, there are methods of achieving resilience.

This chapter looks at mental health exercises that can be adopted to enable patients to regain their emotional equilibrium and a renewed sense of purpose and motivation. Far from being academic recommendations, they are tried and tested and are the successful ones from a process of elimination.

There is an old Yiddish saying that states, "When you are a worm in a jar of horseradish, the world looks horseradish." In other words, when you are in a horrible place in your life, there is a tendency only to see only horrible things around you.

In the 1970s, Aaron T. Beck, an American psychiatrist, regarded as the father of cognitive behavioral therapy, wrote two major publications:

Cognitive Therapy and the Emotional Disorders (Beck 1976) and *Cognitive Therapy of Depression* (Beck 1979). In these, he makes a link between people's psychological problems as presented to the psychotherapist and their perception and understanding, or cognition, of their world.

Beck's basic premise: "When a person's beliefs are overly negative and/or unrealistic about an event, she may be sufficiently disturbed to develop a psychological disorder such as anxiety, depression, or obsessive compulsive behaviour" (Palmer and Dryden 1995). I have shown in part II that obsessive, compulsive, or phobic behaviors such as these can indeed start to take hold as you wrestle with the long-term physical reality of the condition.

Embracing Positive Thinking

More precisely, Beck went on to draw conclusions, with particular emphasis on depression, about the link between people's negative emotions and their negative thinking. One of the aims of cognitive behavioral therapy (CBT), a highly influential and widely used therapy by integrated counsellors and psychotherapists today, is to identify people's negative automatic thoughts, which are given the acronym NATs. It is a good acronym, as it suggests that, like their insect namesakes, gnats, these negative automatic thoughts are small, dark, annoying, and extremely bothersome in large numbers.

It is estimated that we have somewhere between twelve and fifty thousand thoughts per day, of which 80 percent are estimated to be negative and as much as 98 percent are the same thoughts as the previous day (Hawthorne 2014). So our thinking is often ruled by habitual negative thought patterns, whether we realize it or not.

Sitting in the health center waiting to be called in for a blood test, I could not help overhearing an older couple one row behind who were talking aloud to each other. I am sure they did not appreciate that everything they said came across as negative—everything from the weather, to their daughter's shortfalls as a mother, to their teenage grandson's behavior, which all came in for fervent criticism. My psychotherapist's ear heard not one positive remark, no quarter given to understanding or compassion, and I found myself immensely grateful when eventually my name was called for my appointment. It reminded me that such censure, although almost certainly unwitting, could be having an immensely detrimental impact on their own sense of happiness and satisfaction with their lives and the lives of their close family and associates. Negative thoughts are like pebbles thrown into a pond; the ripples spread outward.

As the old Yiddish quote implies, because you are in the grip of a difficult and challenging illness, it is very easy to allow this to influence negatively your whole outlook on life and for it to color your sense of reality and skew your normal judgment. Those with a fear of driving, for example, especially if this is triggered by a bad experience in the car, "put the likelihood of being involved in a crash at 80 percent, whereas the statistical probability is less than one in one hundred thousand" (Sanders and Wills 2005).

Cognitive behavioral therapy recognizes that when a negative frame of mind dominates, people are much more likely to do the following:

- Overestimate the likelihood of further negative events.
- Overestimate long-term negative outcomes, known as catastrophizing
- Underestimate the likelihood of positive solutions.
- Underestimate their ability to cope and apply personal resilience

The first port of call is to recognize how much NATs are invading your thinking. When counselling, I ask clients to count how many times a day they catch themselves thinking negatively, then to write it down and to bring the running daily totals back to me the following week. You can do the same, catching your thoughts each day, writing down the numbers during the day, and adding them up to make an assessment after seven days.

Negative thoughts for the chronically ill may include the following:

- Name-calling: *I am hopeless; I am stupid; I look terrible.*
- Labelling: *I am unlucky; I am lost; I am a burden.*
- Self-blaming: *He looks cross; it must be my fault. I must have done something to upset him. I have messed up.*
- Generalizing: *I can't do anything; I am completely useless.*
- Magnification: *I have forgotten my one appointment; I must be losing my mind.*

- Negative conjecture (what ifs): *What if this (or that) dreadful thing happens?*
- Unrealistic expectations: *I should have; why can't I just …? If only I could.*
- False imperatives: *I must, I ought, and I have to.*
- Negative retrofitting: *If only I had not …*
- Black-and-white thinking: *I am a total failure; I will never rebound.*
- Crystal ball gazing: *There is no point trying this therapy. It won't work; nothing works.*
- Terminal thinking: *I'm finished; I've had enough; I'm through.*
- Catastrophizing: *There's nothing left for me. My life is over; I might as well die.*

(With reference to *Common Thinking Biases*, by Sanders and Wills, 2005)

I could almost guarantee the look of shock on my clients' faces when they returned the following week. Their surprise was because until they started to catch themselves and keep a running total, they had no idea how many times a day they were being negative. Initially, had they been asked, they would probably have identified themselves as taking a fairly balanced view of day-to-day events. In their initial session, they may even have been unable to identify anything that they had a particular problem with in their lives, yet they found themselves inexplicably unhappy and depressed. So understanding the degree of negative prejudice in their whole outlook can come as a huge revelation.

Although having that realization is often groundbreaking in itself, clients may still not know what to do about it. It is quite usual when a negative mind-set is dominant to see the problem as unfixable and to see no way out. "People we see in therapy describe their problems as seemingly intractable, incomprehensible, unending" (Sanders and Wills 2005).

With complete justification and profound understanding, negative thinking may of course be triggered by illness and certainly by lupus in all its forms. Lupus can be so frightening, challenging, and unforgiving that totally understandably, it can often seem insurmountable. Also, as previously argued, sudden feelings of dark depression are a distinctive chemical symptom of lupus flares; I have tracked that the quality of my mood is often susceptible to mini-flares.

Experience has taught me that these feelings will pass along with the physical symptoms. Horsewhisper from the Lupus UK forum wrote movingly to me about this phenomenon: "When I have a flare, it is the feeling of utter despair that gets me: like I'm falling down a rabbit hole … and I don't know when I will stop falling … After the flare, the feeling of despair feels [as if] it was just a dream."

For the benefit of our general mental health, generalized negative constructs about lupus should be challenged and reassurance found in the following facts:

- There are mild, moderate, and severe forms; and people can and do recover from severe to mild.
- Mild to moderate lupus can be well controlled by medication.
- Many with mild forms do not experience any organ involvement.
- When organs are involved, many repair options are available.
- Flares do happen, but what goes up can also come down.
- Flares can be brought under control.
- Flares can reduce in frequency and severity.
- You can learn how to handle your condition better.
- You have recovered from flares before, and there is every possibility that you will do so again.
- The condition can and does go into remission.
- The vast majority of those diagnosed live normal life spans.
- There is the possibility of new treatments and medical advances.

Cognitive behavioral therapy believes that our internal dialogue directly influences how we feel, but these thoughts should first be recognized and then challenged. The approach can be summarized in Thubten Chodron's words: "Don't believe everything you think."

Having identified the thoughts and challenged them, the next step is to change them for ideas that are more positive. It is a fundamental principle of cognitive behavioral therapy that thoughts can be changed and altering them will have a beneficial impact on your overall emotional well-being, such that the ripples on the pond are positive rather than detrimental.

For the second week, I ask clients to stop every time they catch themselves thinking something negative and replace it with something constructive and positive. Affirming phrases begin with "I am":

- *I am resilient.*
- *I am strong.*
- *I am rebuilding.*
- *I am wanted.*
- *I am loved.*
- *I am safe.*

Proactive phrases similarly challenge self-limiting beliefs:

- *I am finding new ways to cope.*
- *I am discovering fresh ways to move forward with my life.*
- *I have changed successfully before; now I am changing again.*

Call center employees are trained to use words ending in *-ly* to create a sense of enthusiastic, supportive intention in their interactions with clients: "I will sort that out for you immediately" or "I totally understand your problem." Analysis shows that the addition of the extra-positive language makes the call center employee seem much more engaged with the clients, on their side, and makes them appear much more trustworthy. You can power up you own positive self-talk using the same technique: "Even though I have lupus …"

- *I absolutely believe that I am improving.*
- *I am moving forward confidently.*
- *I live peacefully and joyfully.*
- *I am completely surrounded by love and support.*

This idea of "powering up" your internal dialogue brings us to an important point about the amount of energy that you invest in these new positive phrases and in applying the methodology. For example, I have encountered reluctance to believe that something apparently so simple can truly alter fundamental mental health, in which case people may be predisposed to be half-hearted in their practice, saying, "I tried that positive self-talk stuff, and it didn't work for me."

In these circumstances, I ask clients to take a moment to cast their minds back to the last thing they worried about, probably within the last two weeks, and to remember how much energy they put into that worry and how often they thought about it. With a typical "mental monologue" or "negative self-talk" (Palmer and Dryden 1995), people will often concentrate on the negative idea intensely and it will repeat in their minds obsessively. It will go round and round, and round again. The more intractable the problem seems, the more it will be revisited. Once this realization is at the forefront of the client's mind, you can ask him to now appreciate the level of intention and commitment that is required to embed the new, positive approach. Handled correctly, this can be something of an "aha" moment.

Self-Criticism

Another aspect of the same problem is the severity with which people self-criticize and simply do not appreciate how tough they are being. In their heads, they will talk to themselves in a way that they would never dream of speaking to another human being. It is a basic counselling methodology to say the following:

- "So what do you say to yourself when that happens?"
- "Did you? Did you really call yourself that?"
- "Now tell me, if another person was as sick as you, would you speak to them like that?"
- "If you knew what they had gone through recently, would you talk to them that way?"
- "If you knew how much pain they were suffering, which of course you do, would you really say that to them? Really, would you?"

Asking clients to switch positions and put themselves in another pair of shoes is usually accompanied by an instant realization that they would apply sensitivity and compassion instead. This is ideally followed by a full appreciation that they are being unduly hard on themselves.

If there is further resistance, then you can ask them to imagine that they are talking to themselves as a sick little girl, sick little boy, or using their first name:

- "Would you talk to your little self like that?"
- "To little [client's first name]: Even if they were going through even a bit of what you have experienced, would you really? No, you would not, would you? I would even go so far as to say *never!*"

The bottom line is that you are experiencing a cruel enough time dealing with lupus; why add to your difficulties by being your own worst critic? If anyone needs a friend right now, it is you. If anyone needs a kind supporter right now, it is undoubtedly you.

It is crucial that you understand the power of your intention and have confidence that this new daily process of replacing negative phrases with proactive, reinforcing, and affirmative phrases will, with practice and by degrees, change your internal dialogue.

You should realize that on bad days when pain or stress takes over, your subconscious may dominate and the tendency to regress to old ingrained patterns may increase. Remember, it takes twenty-one days to establish a new habit, so be kind to yourself and appreciate that in compounding terms, every negative thought replaced with a positive is tangible improvement. Given what you are dealing with, you should congratulate yourself on that move forward and that brilliant hard-won progress in the teeth of such adversity!

Nevertheless, in some circumstances, despite every effort, you may struggle to stay positive. I certainly did and still do on down days that can come out of nowhere and trip you up. It is also necessary to appreciate that you may have inherited underlying negative mantras from your family and upbringing that can lie dormant in the subconscious but which can rise unbidden at times of stress and prove unhelpful. An example would be a father's voice saying, "No pain, no gain" or "Life is hard and then you die" (no, seriously, I have come across this one). In these circumstances, at times of acute stress, it is good to have a basic statement that is easy to remember and can be substituted when negative emotions overwhelm.

Research shows that rhyming phrases are more memorable and make a greater emotional impact on the human psyche than plain statements.

There is also evidence that people find that sayings are more convincing and believable if they rhyme, which is why commercial slogans often go down this route to imprint products on our minds. This can also be reinforced by alliteration—that is, repetition of the same first letter, as in "Brown bears are boxing"—and this is another common advertising trick of the trade. My go-to phrase through this lupus journey has been "Every day, in every way, I am getting better and better" (Emile Cove 1857–1926). This simple, perhaps some would say banal, little phrase has been my backstop. Granted, it has been said occasionally through gritted teeth in the face of pain and despite my logical mind intervening with, *Are you serious!*

Nonetheless, I have confidence that it is reaching my subconscious—and what is the alternative? I have experienced catastrophizing, as you have read, and find that this method makes me feel consistently better when that happens. Think of such sayings as safety blankets that can be reached for at points of maximum nervousness.

Furthermore, the principle can be expanded using the inspirational work of Louise Hay and her daily affirmations and positive statements available at https://www.louisehay.com. The affirmations section provides an inexhaustible source of positive self-talk for reading or for audio download. You can peruse these and find ones that speak to you and you can write these or any of the positive phrases discussed down on small cards or on sticky notes, putting them in places that you go to regularly until they are embedded.

Rebuilding your Sense of Purpose

"What do you do?" This is a standard social opening question, and many of us are defined by our jobs and tasks in life. Our defined roles provide a daily framework and a plan for our future. They can be inextricably linked to our status and sense of fulfilment. A serious illness can bring our jobs and even our basic household tasks to a halt, making us unable to function as we used to, but it goes deeper. This need for a purpose in life is profound and is fundamental to our need to get ahead and improve our lives and the lives of our family. Human beings are naturally project orientated. We are the ultimate toolmakers.

In striking contrast to the primates, from which we evolved, "the human hand has a much larger, more muscular, mobile and fully opposable thumb combined with fingers that have shortened and straightened" (Young 2003). Anthropologists have long argued that the additional capabilities and dexterity that this brings is the basis for our superior advancement as a species, combined of course with bipedalism and large brains: "Our fully opposable thumbs enabled our ancestors to make tools which conquered the world" (Fecht 2015). She goes on to argue that the wraparound fist that the configuration also gives to the human hand was also an advantage for success in fights, but I digress. The crucial point to make is that the ability to apply ourselves to projects is ingrained in our psyches. Therefore, because we are naturally task orientated, a sense of achievement can be critical to our mental well-being.

Debilitating illness can stop this beneficial process, making you unable to work normally or as you used to. Rhythms are broken, and plans taken for granted are overturned. This can rob you of a sense of purpose, and without your usual tasks, you can struggle to regain meaning and reframe your life.

This is particularly challenging when you have an unpredictable condition such as lupus. Lupus, with its flares and mini-flares, can be especially difficult to control. This lack of any sense of being able to plot a course can make you feel rudderless at sea.

The first healthy thing to acknowledge is that that healing in general is not usually a precise process with a line on the graph following a neat trajectory from bottom left to top right. It is also a highly individual process: "No two persons have the same mind or the same body" (Swami Vivekananda).

You should become comfortable with the idea that your recovery is unlikely to follow a set pattern. Why would it? You will appreciate that healing is rarely sequential. If you know that it is quite usual for progress to be made despite being apparently random from a day-to-day perspective, you will be much less dejected and disappointed by setbacks. You will know that this is quite normal. A golfing professional once pointed out to me, "Your scorecard is not a picture book."

In other words, what matters at the end of the day is that you get from the tee to the green in the fewest number of shots, but if you are bunkered or in the rough several times and yet come out of them successfully, your scorecard will not reveal this. So don't expend energy worrying about how things *should be* moving forward because such a manual does not exist for lupus; there is no such thing. Nor is this an examination in which your workings are judged. Recognize that this is healing and healing can be messy but no less valid. This relieves the human psyche profoundly, especially if you have perfectionist or competitive tendencies.

Furthermore, you would not expect to stop a supertanker on a sixpence. So a complex disease such as lupus, which impacts multiple bodily functions, may well take time to slow down and to get under control. Appreciate this and straightaway you take the pressure off yourself to secure a "textbook" recovery.

There may be watersheds, and what begins as a temporary pause in symptoms may, over a series of weeks, become more enduring. This can be accompanied by small advances in functioning, and over time these little improvements can accumulate to become much more than the sum of their individual parts.

Patients should look to accept these increments in a relaxed manner, ultimately reaching an improved level of health. Many lupus patients like me will have been walking around for years with undiagnosed symptoms. I concluded that with the flare under control, I would be in a better position than at any time in my adult life because the medication and the knowledge would be in place to manage my condition correctly. This was my journey's destination but at that point, both physically and psychologically, sight of the harbor was still distant. So what more could be done?

Following Beck's groundbreaking work in the 1970s, cognitive behaviorists have expanded the therapy into creating constructive answers for many kinds of psychological problems and emotional difficulties. Having identified the negative thoughts, challenged them, and devised a new positive internal dialogue, modern cognitive behavioral therapy then goes on to form a collaborative alliance with the client to break her problems down into achievable solutions. This therapeutic approach involves setting targets, creating agendas, keeping diaries, agreeing on goals, doing homework on those goals, and measuring improvement against those targets.

At this point, I can feel you reeling at the sheer impossibility of applying anything so structured to lupus, with its level of uncertainty. "Isn't that like trying to take a cup of water on a roller coaster?" I hear you say.

Well, there are indeed aspects of the approach that I have found to be very useful. Yes, they must be adapted to suit, but I have proved to myself that it can offer constructive answers to some of the seemingly intractable problems that the condition presents: "We must be willing to let go of the life we've planned so as to have the life waiting for us" (Joseph Campbell).

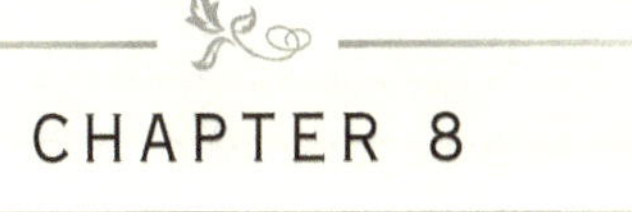

CHAPTER 8

The Power of Little Steps

The man who moved a mountain began by carrying away small stones.
—Chinese proverb

Fundamental to this recommended approach is the idea of breaking progress down into steps. Little steps allow you to minimize any sense of stress and to maximize your sense of achievement. Recovery from serious illness is best done gradually. This is not only acceptable but is in fact an optimum way for the body and the mind to regain their strength.

In practice, our lives are built on daily tasks. The mundane is actually the foundation of the majority of our achievements, whatever the size, and there is an old Zen Buddhist saying that recognizes this: "Before enlightenment, chop wood, carry water. After enlightenment, chop wood, carry water."

I too used to have tiers of priorities and have short-, medium-, and long-term goals, but now that my energy was utterly diminished and completely unreliable, a new system was required, one that accommodated variable focus, variable energy, and variable physical capacity. It also needed in-built flexibility to allow for good days and bad days, and it was quite clear that I was going to have to start small!

Rebuilding a Sense of Purpose

Lists had always been part of my daily and weekly process, but they were lists often achieved with assistants and at least one team working with me. I had always followed one golden rule: If it was on the list, it got done without fail, unless altered by an unavoidable, extenuating circumstance. This might seem blindingly obvious, but I have worked previously with an assistant director who was well known for writing long and detailed lists, none of which he then followed. It probably helped him just to write things down, but it is more dynamic to go further. My new lists were compiled (shakily, as it was difficult to write), with a mix of daily and short-term tasks that were not time limited. Taking out the time pressure allowed me to work with my body rather than forcing it in any way.

Even the simplest things were put on the list, such as unstack the dishwasher and fold clothing, because these can all be hugely difficult to achieve if severely ill. It took some eight months of bed and sofa rest before I could attempt unstacking the dishwasher. Then every piece of crockery had to be carried with two hands to ensure that it was not dropped, because my hands were stiff and shaking, and handled one by one so as not to strain the joints in my thumbs and wrists. Even then, I sent a couple of pieces of china spinning across the kitchen floor to their demise. The first time I managed to restack, my husband, who had been in charge for months, rearranged several items to his preferred method. I got tearful because the process of bending down and up had been so painful and exhausting that I simply could not cope with the speed with which he had redone all my hard work.

Completing the tasks, however small, allowed me the huge satisfaction of ticking them off the list. Uncompleted tasks were never dropped, merely carried forward, but crucially, all, even the tiniest, were eventually done. As the days went by, I took satisfaction from a little ruled notebook of ticked tasks that grew and grew.

Your tasks may be larger and more complex, such as driving the children to school, running errands, and answering multiple emails. You may take them for granted and say that they don't count and don't matter. But you must look at them in the context of how much effort they really cost you to achieve with your lupus, especially on a bad day.

You need to accommodate days when simply nothing but the basics of eating, taking your medication, and washing can be achieved. This is exactly why the lists are designed to be on a can-do basis only and are not time limited in any way. Most importantly, what they do start to chip away at is the sense that you are unable to achieve anything meaningful, which merely builds a feeling of powerlessness in the face of a great mountain of "the not done."

David Allen, in his *New York Times* best seller *Getting Things Done*, identifies what he calls "amorphous blobs of undo-ability" and notes that "any would, could, or should held only in the psyche creates irrational and unresolvable pressure" (Allen 2015). He sees lists as the starting point to breaking down seemingly impossible tasks.

While recognizing that Allen teaches incredibly busy professionals how to tackle seemingly insurmountable large-scale projects, my endeavors seemed no less challenging and large-scale with lupus. He clearly states, "I have discovered over the years the practical value of working on personal productivity improvement from the bottom up, starting with the most mundane, ground-floor level of current activity and commitments." Therefore, the fact that my mundane lists were my entire compass was irrelevant. What was important was they pushed back in tiny increments against a terrible sense of failure. As time progressed, my lists began to anchor me in a sea of uncertainty.

Rebuilding a Sense of Achievement

> When times are tough and we lose confidence in ourselves. No
> other creature on earth has the capacity to redefine itself. We do.
> —Deepak Chopra

Much media is devoted to the big picture, to highlighting ambitious life goals and to long-term achievements. People follow celebrities who travel extensively and pursue global ambitions. For someone with a chronic health condition, this can all seem discouraging unless she is able to reframe it in some way. With my restricted compass, of particular impact were the seasonal expectations of Easter, the summer holidays, Halloween, and Christmas. It is so easy to feel totally dislocated from the rhythms of normal life when very ill, which can make you compromise or simply not be able to take part fully in many of these traditional cycles. In 2012, I narrowly avoided being hospitalized on Christmas Eve.

If you are usually a "doer," you will take the ability to multitask entirely for granted. "The tidying can wait" is actually a foreign concept to the majority of modern women juggling private lives and jobs. Well, with this condition, you will need to park that concept, as it will be much healthier for you to break your day back down into its component parts and abandon any guilt about some ideal level of achievement.

A Diary

You will need a diary that contains those appointments or visits that are time specific. Depending on the degree to which you suffer from lupus fog, you may need someone close to keep an eye on your appointments for you to ensure that you don't miss them.

Then, to rebuild your sense of purpose and achievement, in line with cognitive behavioral therapeutic principles, I suggest that you run two lists alongside your diary. The rest of your life should be orientated into these two lists. No distinction is made between so-called leisure pursuits and tasks or necessities on these two lists. Everything simply comes under the presumption "to be done."

A Macro List and a Daily Tasks List

Fundamental to the idea behind the two lists is that while they are an excellent start, it is possible to rebuild a greater sense of purpose by going beyond daily tasks to setting goals. These two lists are therefore separated into a macro goals list and a daily tasks list that also includes micro-goals. Therefore, in summary, you have the following:

- A diary—time-sensitive appointments and arrangements
- A macro list—a list of broader goals and targets (five items or more per goal)
- A daily tasks list—contains both daily tasks and micro-goals

Goal Characteristics

Overall, the three crucial characteristics of all goals, whether macro or micro, are that they encompass the following:

- Incorporate both physical and mental challenges
- Are gentle on the body
- Are not time pressured

Pacing Yourself

For those with lupus, whatever system is set in motion, it is crucial to accommodate the inherent unpredictability of the medical condition itself but also of the individual healing process. If you build in time limits, then there is a danger that you will prioritize the deadline instead of listening to your body. It is so important to rest when tired, irrespective of when that is; whether fifteen minutes after starting, half an hour in, or two hours later, the body must come first.

Understanding your limits is a building block of the healing process. There is often a desire to use up all the available energy on tasks, given that this is the norm for well people. Indeed, in this pressurized modern era, it is perhaps stating the obvious to say that many overextend their energies and are rest deficient. When coping with chronic illness, you should build in recuperation and healing time. You should be hypervigilant as to the needs of your body, bear witness to any changes, and be alert to your warning signs.

You must learn to pace yourself, but this can be tremendously hard. Firstly, because let's face it: being ill can be boring. Secondly, because frustration can make you overdo it. Thirdly, there is a compulsion when you feel better to fit in all the things that you want to either do or think you ought to be doing. This is why it is so important to create a list of intellectually nourishing things to do when you are recuperating.

Through trial and error to determine what worked best for me, I began to follow the principle of spending about one-third of my time on the tasks or chores that I wanted to do in order to avoid severe payback pain and fatigue. This methodology then left one-third for recuperation with stimulating pursuits (which we examine in more detail shortly) and one-third for healing with sleep or meditating. This became the template for pacing my activities. It overrode any mental chatter about what I thought I ought to be achieving and any emotional feelings of guilt. Furthermore, once established as a principle, family and friends would help police my activity levels and tell me to sit down and rest when they assessed that I was getting carried away and doing too much.

This is also why the bulk of your planning and organizing, aside from the diary, needs to be open-ended and unscheduled. On this basis, the goals will, in essence, do no harm because they are flexible and adaptive to good days and bad days; they accept that improvement may be nonlinear. If the micro-goals are not completed one day, they are simply carried forward, always working within the basic principle that small steps are best. Small steps pose the least risk of overdoing it, while still giving a direction of travel and ultimately a sense of achievement.

The in-built flexibility becomes your friend and an essential part of your healing process. The system is designed to harness both the mind and the body and to benefit both. It is essential that you write these goals down, preferably in a series of small books or pads designed specifically for taking notes. You might choose reporter's ruled notebooks or something less utilitarian and with a meaningful or uplifting design that helps you celebrate your activities a little more. Whatever style you are drawn to, it is essential that you write them down. In this era of technology, you may prefer to record them on a tablet or a phone, which is acceptable, but it is imperative that you have a means of ticking off the tasks as they are completed.

<u>Setting Goals</u>

Dr. Gail Matthews, PhD, a professor of psychology at the Dominican University of California, completed research into goal setting and its impact on achievement. She split a group of 267 participants from around the world—including entrepreneurs, educators, health-care professionals, artists, attorneys, bankers, marketers, human services providers, managers, vice presidents, and directors of nonprofits—into those who thought about their goals and those who wrote down their goals. She discovered that those that wrote them down accomplished considerably more than those who did not—in fact, some 50.1 percent more. This improvement purely from writing down goals underlines the mental and motivational importance of something that might otherwise be taken for granted. It is not to be dismissed. Indeed, it is an essential building block of reframing your life and your sense of satisfaction in that life.

Writing down a list of higher-level macro goals can start to frame your activities in the simplest of ways. For example, if your lupus is so severe that you are forced to spend a great deal of time recuperating, then you can, in this era of multimedia, organize this greatly. For example, you may be keen on particular sports and can focus on these. Personally, always a fan of cricket and tennis, I made a point of following my favorite teams and individual players in a structured way. In tennis, I would systematically follow the Grand Slam tournaments, the Australian Open, the French Open, Wimbledon, and the US Open; and when it came to the 2012 Olympics held in the UK, I had a specific goal, which was to view all the British gold medals live. In the end, I managed all except one, that elusive shooting gold, but caught a replay later so little was lost.

Using the television, a tablet, and audio, you can pursue macro and micro-goals and work your way through topics that you find interesting. You might take the opportunity to learn a great deal more about a particular period in history or about wildlife, view those movies that won Best Picture at the Oscars, read the works of one particular author, or listen to audiobooks along the same principle. Music goals can be included, with specific genres and artists followed. Janet, my great friend at university, had the complete set of Beethoven's nine symphonies on her shelf.

So much is now almost instantly at our disposal, despite being bedridden or housebound. The rule of thumb is that it must be a series or a set of five or more things to count as a macro goal. In this time of media abundance, the world's creativity and knowledge is at your fingertips. The overall aim is the sense of an absorbing project that can be pursued over a series of days or weeks. Completing phases in the project then gives a sense of progress.

Achieving Absorption

Using distraction as a means of pain relief is widely reported. The idea is to stimulate nerves in another part of the brain to those that are being activated by the pain.

In 2011, experiments into electronic gaming as a distraction highlighted that the level of absorption and participation in the gaming as opposed to passive television watching improved the level of pain relief: "Participants in both experiments had significantly higher pain tolerance and reported less pain with the active distraction compared with passive or no distraction" (Jameson 2011). In other words, the more stimulating the distraction, the more helpful it may be with chronic pain. The possibilities of pain relief aside, getting absorbed mentally and emotionally in your projects and goals will add to your sense of satisfaction and purpose. This is sometimes described as an ability to get lost in a task.

Avoiding Depressing Influences

The one caveat to make is to be wary of deeply negative storylines or dark extended plots, as these can dampen your mood when you are already vulnerable. It is an old Fleet Street saying that "if it bleeds, it leads," so also be aware that journalism, both on the television and in print, is apt to emphasize the negative to attract our attention.

After studying reactions on the cerebral cortex, which demonstrated a greater increase in electrical activity in reaction to miserable and alarming news compared to neutral or positive tales, Tiffany A. Ito concluded that the brain is more stimulated by negative stories than positive news (Ito 1998). She and her team proposed that this "negative bias" stemmed from the time when our evolutionary survival depended on us noticing danger early.

Laughter

An extension of this warning, and one of the best pieces of advice given to me by my friend Juliet, was to make room for laughter despite serious illness. Dr. Annette Goodheart, in her comprehensive book *Laughter Therapy*, writes, "As a therapist, I've had thousands of hours of experience working with people suffering from minor ailments and terminal illnesses, including cancer, AIDS, MS, and arthritis; I have worked with anorexics, survivors of sexual abuse, and the suicidally depressed. The good news is that laughter is a powerful healing force. It's not a panacea, but it can be part of any programme for healing physically, emotionally, or spiritually" (Goodheart 1994).

So make sure that within this system of viewing and reading, you include humor and comedy, whether this is books, boxed sets, or movies—basically, whatever tickles your particular sense of humor and really makes you laugh. Not just smile but laugh, preferably out loud. Deep laughter that moves the chest, expands the diaphragm, and exercises the breathing muscles is ideal and combats long periods of enforced rest. It will bring more oxygen into the bloodstream, thereby lifting you physically and releasing feel-good endorphins in the brain. Remember, "He who laughs, lasts" (Mary Pettibone Poole).

The essential thing is to write down your goal of watching, for example, series I, II, and III on the higher-level macro goal list, and then breaking it down as micro-goals on the smaller daily lists.

There were tasks that I would like to have done, but they put too much strain on my wrists and finger joints to be sustainable. This included knitting, sewing, and embroidery. You may be able to pick these things up and put them down satisfactorily, and the movement may prove beneficial rather than painful. You can try it and see.

As we have seen from the gaming research, activities should be mentally, emotionally, and, where possible, physically stimulating. For example, having been sent book details by Hay House of the cathartic results of tidying and space clearing, by Denise Linn, I set myself the macro-level task of tidying all the mid-height drawers and cupboards in the house. So I wrote down my higher level goal as "tidy the bedroom drawers," and then it was broken down into micro-goals on the daily lists, as in "dressing table; chest drawers one, two, and three; side tables one and two," and each one was then ticked off on completion.

I could sit down while doing the drawers. The movements were not repetitive, and the contents were not heavy, so the drawers were a good place to start. My normal schedule would not have had the room to devote to such small, mundane tasks. Therefore, on completion, I gained satisfaction from everything now being in its rightful place, all clean and up to date. There was even, on occasion, added pleasure from finding items that had been lost for ages.

Sometimes it could take me over three weeks to tidy one single drawer, but tidy them I did, one by one. Completing tasks over successive days or weeks was satisfying, giving a steadily improving sense of achievement. This simple process can gradually help to rebuild your shattered sense of purpose.

Asking for Help

Both lists should also be open to containing another feature, which is the "get help with" aspect. When you train as a counsellor and psychotherapist, you are assessed in depth, and indeed continuous self-examination and self-awareness are an essential part of the job. One of my characteristics had been identified early on as "overt self-reliance"—in other words, a tendency to be highly independent and reluctant to ask for help. Addison Dean was diagnosed with lupus at age twenty-two, and on her blog, she describes embarrassment at not being able to do things for herself and about how difficult it is getting used to asking for the help she needs.

You need to practically and sensibly appreciate that some tasks will simply not get done without cooperation, and this feature embraces that reality. For example, well-judged requests for help with lifting heavy items or unscrewing tops will ultimately allow you to achieve more without setting you back. Although I would be the first to recognize that guilt and embarrassment about having to ask for help are totally understandable, you need to park these negative feelings in order to make the best progress.

Furthermore, it is easy for everyone involved to feel as if they are treading on eggshells. Your concern for the feelings of your loved ones and friends should be assuaged because they are likely to be relieved if they know that you will come to them when needed, rather them having to worry in silence that you may be overdoing it.

A macro list might look as follows:

Macro List

- Tidy kitchen utensil drawers
- Follow Wimbledon tennis
- Read new author
- Find new morning stretching exercises on YouTube

- Get help organizing photos
- Get help washing and drying the blankets
- Order new clothes

Remember, there is no distinction between necessary chores and tasks and recuperation pursuits; they all implicitly come under the heading "To be done."

Daily List

The daily list contains both daily tasks and micro-goals. It contains things you hope to realistically start and complete that day, depending on how you feel when you wake up, but recognizing that this might change and some things will therefore be carried over into second, third, or even fourth days. Several times, it took me weeks to complete the tidying of one set of drawers because I was having such a difficult time with debilitating symptoms. Again, there is no distinction between leisure and necessity.

- Unstack the dishwasher
- Tidy left-hand side kitchen drawers one, two, and three
- Watch tennis match
- Read chapters one and two
- Get help putting the gray blanket back on
- Order repeat prescription
- Order two new T-shirts online
- Invite X for coffee

When tasks and or goals are completed, tick off all component parts, the kitchen drawers one, two, and three, for example. You may query why it is recommended that you tick off each individual task when completed. Well, it is important because this pedantic method is a process of reinforcement of the amount of things that you are actually doing each day, not what you think you might be achieving, which will probably seem much less.

You will remember when we looked at the principle of a negative outlook that it is easy to fall into the trap of focusing on what you are not doing rather than what you are doing. This seemingly simple process blocks that negative mind-set and instead builds a realization that you are contributing and making concrete progress every day. "Take the first step in faith. You don't have to see the whole staircase. Just take the first step" (Martin Luther King Jr.).

Furthermore, as the days go by, you will begin to appreciate roughly how much you can achieve on a good day and how much is overdoing it. You will then have the data to rein back on the second and third days if necessary. Clearly, it is not an exact science because lupus can upset plans at short notice, but as Mark Victor Hansen noted, "There will always be challenges, obstacles, and less-than-perfect conditions. So what."

This is a process backed by tried-and-tested psychotherapeutic methods tailored to lupus. These deceptively straightforward techniques can harness your natural curiosity and reawaken your creativity. They can push back against negative feelings of boredom, frustration, and uselessness, thereby rebuilding your sense of purpose and achievement. It is suggested that you apply this system diligently for twenty-one days, then note if there is marked change in your outlook and a positive shift in your consciousness.

CHAPTER 9

Harnessing the Breath and Mindfulness

Your breathing is so ordinary, so mundane, that its
true significance can easily pass you by.
—Dr. Danny Penman, *The Art of Breathing*

Breath Work

The importance of breath work became apparent to me in 2013, when suffering from tightness across my diaphragm that felt like a band being tensioned by invisible hands. One of my helpful community nurses pointed out that my breathing had probably become shallow due to sitting curved forward on a sofa or in bed for over a year. I also read that opioid pain relief can reduce the depth of normal respiration.

Her words reminded me of some yoga classes that I had taken, where we had been instructed that most people do not breathe properly. We had been given an exercise where we took deep breaths, filled our lungs, and pulled the air right down into our stomachs such that they expanded outward, before expelling it noisily. So when the restriction began across my rib cage, I started to breathe more deeply in this manner and found that it made me more relaxed. Little did I know at the time that I had embarked on a basic tenet of non-drug-related lupus treatment, namely breath work.

It is indeed much more normal for people to breathe shallowly, particularly women, for whom the idea of expanding the stomach goes against the cosmetic and cultural desire for flatness in this area. So they contain their breathing to their chest instead. This reduced breathing brings less oxygen into the lungs, certainly to the lower levels, and this lack of oxygen distresses the body. The human mind then feels more tension. Therefore, learning to breathe properly is a fundamental building block of many relaxation exercises because it slows down the heartbeat and reduces blood pressure.

Breathing deeply and calmly has been shown to dramatically reduce the fight-or-flight adrenalin response that makes the physical body highly stressed. In the 1970s, cardiologist Dr. Herbert Benson identified a need to instigate what he called the "relaxation response" as a direct alternative. His analysis showed that instead of this extreme response being usefully triggered by genuine danger and life-threatening situations, in fact the stresses and strains of the modern world is instigating the emergency response far too often.

This in turn is provoking medical conditions such as cardiovascular disease, adrenal fatigue, gastrointestinal ailments, and insomnia, which are all high stress related. Dr. Benson's landmark book *The Relaxation Response* recommended a range of techniques to offset the fight-or-flight response and the promotion of relaxation instead. His recommended starting point is ten to twenty minutes per day of practicing deep breathing and relaxing all the muscles. Dr. Benson profoundly believed in the importance of mind and body relaxation to physical health, and he went on to establish the Mind Body Medical Institute at Massachusetts General Hospital in Boston.

Mindfulness

> If the future seems overwhelming, remember
> that it comes one moment at a time.
> —Beth Mende Conny

As we have noted, the introduction of functional magnetic resonance imaging (fMRI) in the 1990s has allowed scientists to study brain activity and function to a completely different level of detail and accuracy. They have been able to discover that far from steadily deteriorating over time, as previously thought, that instead certain activities and experiences can be beneficial for the brain. They have been able to look at people suffering from stress and to note the negative effect of cortisol on brain function. Significantly, they have also been able to conclude that practicing mindfulness, even for as little as eight weeks, has a positive effect on the brain.

The philosophical roots of mindfulness reach back over 2,500 years into the fundamentals of Buddhism and Hinduism, as well as Taoism and Sufism. The first mindfulness teacher of the modern era was Thich Nhat Hanh, a Vietnamese monk who wished to give his people, who had been devastated by the Vietnam War, the tools to survive and rebuild when they had lost everything. The use of mindfulness for chronic psychological and physical conditions continues to expand, and I have found it to be very beneficial in coping with lupus.

Concentration on the breath is the foundation stone of mindfulness, and I have employed the following simple breathing exercise as my first port of call on the onset of pain, anxiety, or stress. You might try it the next few times that you experience such situations to see if it can be helpful to you too.

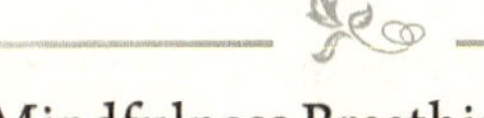

Mindfulness Breathing Exercise

To practice mindfulness at its most basic, find a space where you will be quiet and not interrupted. You should wear comfortable nonrestrictive clothing. You do not have to sit in any particular pose. Indeed, for lupus patients it is valuable to be as comfortable as possible, probably with your back and legs supported by soft pillows on a sofa or a bed so as not to put any additional strain on joints and muscles, with your legs likely raised and with your hands gently resting on your thighs or in your lap.

As relaxation spreads, your body temperature is inclined to drop, especially if you have a chronic illness, so it is best to wrap yourself in a soft blanket or shawl and to make sure your feet are warm. Place the tip of your tongue behind your front teeth, as this relaxes the throat and the neck, but don't worry if you forget. The idea is not to create any tension on your muscles, so the default position is not to force anything and to adopt whatever feels most comfortable.

Close your eyes, focusing your attention inward. At its most simplistic, mindfulness practice just focuses on the breath going in and out. Do not try to control the breath; simply experience it coming cold into the nose, travelling cold down the esophagus, expanding the stomach like a small balloon, and then experience the air expelling back up through your chest and escaping warmly out of the mouth. If you forget to breathe out through your mouth, don't worry. Notice instead how it feels cold on the way into your nose and warm on the way out. Hear the whooshing sound between your ears as the breath is drawn in and out, in and out, and as you sink back farther, feel the softness of your pillows, sofa, or bed behind and beneath you. Relax.

You are fully supported now, feeling calm and safe, and your stomach may gurgle as you start to relax more fully. If thoughts start to come into your mind, let them pass through like clouds across the sky. Acknowledge them but do not engage with them. Let them pass gently on—there they go—and then return to your breath. Place one hand on your stomach so that you can feel the air filling the stomach and expanding it and then going down … expanding … and then going down.

Slowly breathe—take your time; there is no rush—in and out, in and out. There is no system, no rules. Simply focus on the breath as you relax more and more, further and further, just on the air coming in and out, in and out—feeling calm and safe, deeply relaxed. If a thought intrudes, acknowledge it but don't engage. Let it pass gently on. Breathing steadily, you may start to feel a little light-headed, but not unpleasantly so. Pause at any time if you feel that you are starting to hyperventilate or are uncomfortable.

Then, when you feel it is appropriate, take three extra-deep breaths in through your nose and out through your mouth—three deep, purifying breaths—and gently open your eyes, stretch out your fingers, and wriggle your toes. How do you feel? Stretch and wriggle a bit more and then give yourself a minute to appreciate how you feel before getting up slowly. You can use the record function on your phone to talk through this exercise in your own voice and then play it back.

This simple breathing exercise can be used as a first port of call with the onset of pain, panic, or anxiety. It can be used beneficially in combination with medication for pain or anxiety or with other complementary solutions such as essential oils, which will be discussed in more detail in part III.

If all else fails and the onset of pain, panic, or anxiety is sudden and severe, then remember that your first and immediate reaction should be to make one long deep exhale to empty out the lungs. This will then inevitably enforce a deep inhale next, and it may even take a couple of breaths to regain enough oxygen back, which means that you will have adopted deep respiration at the onset of your panic, which is hugely beneficial. You can then continue to breathe deeply, fully in and out, for the next few minutes, and the whole process should help you to feel more centered. If you are in a position to do so, you can place one hand over your stomach to check that you are taking air right down through your body. You can view this as your fallback strategy should you be taken suddenly off guard.

<u>Mindfulness: The Second Stage</u>

The practice of mindfulness extends beyond being aware of the breath and ties in with the work already completed on negative automatic thinking. Dr. Danny Penman notes, "You'll probably spend thirty-six minutes worrying today (most people do)." The process of worrying means that you are looking forward to possibilities and negatively conjecturing about things that might happen but which have not actually taken place. Get this: they may never happen! So you are spending time and energy on a projection. You are getting fearful and stressed over a forecast, when at least ten things may come between that forecast and reality.

Worse than that, your body does not know that it is a projection and reacts to your thoughts in the present tense. Of fundamental importance is that the body does not hear the word *if*, so it gets fearful and stressed, as if these forecasts are current reality.

In 2004, Scott Bishop and his team of clinical psychologists, based primarily at the University of Toronto, sought to clarify the burgeoning field of mindfulness into two distinct phases. The first phase concerned "the somatic sensations of his or her own breathing. Whenever attention wanders from the breath to inevitable thoughts and feelings that arise, the client will simply take notice of them and let them go as attention is returned to the breath" (Bishop 2004), and this is the approach we have already covered.

Then they clarified that the second part of mindfulness is a natural extension of the breathing exercise in that the mind is not allowed to follow, then dwell, and definitely not obsess on "thoughts, worries, or ruminations" (Bishop 2004) that occur throughout the day. Instead, the mind is brought back to focus, as it did on the breath, to "the here and now during the course of the day." Therefore, the original principle is broadened out to encompass all aspects of everyday life.

The *Merriam-Webster Dictionary* defines mindfulness as "the practice of maintaining a non-judgemental state of heightened or complete awareness of one's thoughts, emotions, or experiences on a moment-to-moment basis." John Keats, the famous English romantic poet who suffered from tuberculosis, wrote to his friend Benjamin Bailey in 1817, "I look not for it; if it be not in the present hour—nothing startles me beyond the moment."

Jon Kabat-Zinn was born in 1944, and his background is in molecular biology, with a PhD from the Massachusetts Institute of Technology (MIT). He is a professor emeritus of medicine and founder of the Stress Reduction Clinic and the Center for Mindfulness in Medicine, Health Care, and Society at the University of Massachusetts Medical School in the United States. He developed his mindfulness-based stress reduction program (MSBR) to improve patients' ability to cope with stress, pain, and illness. It is a structured eight-week course based on meditation and hatha yoga. His book *Mindfulness for Beginners: Reclaiming the Present Moment—and Your Life* sets out the basics of his approach. Kabat Zinn also wrote *Full Catastrophe Living (Revised Edition): How to Cope with Stress, Pain, and Illness using Mindfulness Meditation.*

His work first came to my attention in 2013, when, with my trusty small tablet, I was tracking down methods of pain management for those resistant to mainstream drug treatment. I noted that in 1979 he had specifically recruited people who were experiencing chronic pain, with their backs, with cancer, as victims of industrial accidents, and paraplegics for his meditation program. He found that people in chronic pain have an altered relationship with their pain that is non-beneficial. This idea of a "relationship" developing with chronic pain really spoke to me. You will perhaps recall in an earlier chapter that my pain had almost developed a personality of its own, and a hugely difficult one at that.

I read that Kabat-Zinn's mindfulness process allowed his patients to differentiate between their thoughts and their bodily sensations, which led to the important realization that "the pain is not me." This concept immediately appealed because it effectively put emotional space between my chronic pain and me. I realized that I felt responsible for appeasing my pain and was experiencing a sense of failure when I could not. Furthermore, when repeated time and time again, these feelings of failure were turning into frustration and depression. The idea that his methods enabled his patients to develop a healthier relationship with their pain looked very useful.

So moving on from the simple breathing exercise, as explained above, which I actively employed and perfected when the pain started to expand and the anxiety to build, I then began to practice Kabat-Zinn's in-the-moment mindfulness.

This means placing your full attention on the small physical details of daily tasks and happenings. For example, when bathing, eating breakfast, making beverages, or moving around, concentrate on the feel, scents, sights, and sounds of your immediate environment. Instead of the mind wandering ahead of these everyday events, which is the norm—planning, worrying, and obsessing—the attention is brought back to the absolute present. In addition, you should strive to take pleasure in these minutiae.

The overthinking habit may be hard to break at first, and you may well catch yourself mentally multitasking as usual. When this happens, just apply the same method as with those intrusive thoughts in the breath meditation, simply bringing the focus gently back to the present. Acknowledge the thoughts but let them pass. Again, if a negative sensation or idea pops into your head, just acknowledge it without judgment and let it pass.

Over time, the process is said to create a gap between your sensations and your mental reactions, which makes sense because you are perfecting breaking the inevitable link between the two. This, in turn, begins to erode your ingrained response patterns. "Between stimulus and response, there is a space. In that space is our power to choose our response. In our response lies our growth and our freedom" (Viktor Frankl, MD, holocaust survivor).

Finding a way to create this gap is especially important to those suffering from chronic pain, for as Patrizia Collard states, "Without experiencing distance from—for instance—physical or psychological pain, we tend to feel that we are nothing but pain."

Mindfulness does not suppress thoughts and feelings. One of the planks of Kabat-Zinn's approach is to react nonjudgmentally, identifying that we tend to have automatic labels for people and events: "This is bad," "That is a problem," "Such and such is wrong." Instead, he encouraged his patients to be neutral and to acknowledge but not define according to habit. As Gabriel Shaw writes, "Your opinions are not facts."

With repetition, you can learn to stand outside your pain. You will no longer attach negative emotions such as anxiety or guilt to it. If it starts to increase, it will not raise emotional concerns automatically, concerns that just make the experience of pain even worse. Kabat-Zinn's simple process actually breaks down old fearful thinking patterns. It also goes on to impact brain function directly by opening up new neuropathways, and by degrees it retrains and then restimulates our brains.

Thinking in the moment will leave less room for thinking ahead, and fewer negative thoughts will bolster an overall sense of satisfaction. You will develop a sense of delight in little things, and this creates a raft of contentment supporting your day. Remember, it takes twenty-one days to embed a new habit, so be kind to yourself about relapses and keep going with the new thinking. If you get distracted, simply pick up from where you left off.

I began with appreciating any task, however small, which I found easy having gone from a situation of being able to do hardly anything. Lifting a kettle, even two-handed, to avoid putting pressure on my joints and make my own first cup of tea of the day was celebrated as a personal triumph. The countryside outside my door became an unlimited source of delight, as often rising early, surrendering the nightly battle with pain, I would see the dawn creep up over the horizon and hear the chorus of wild birds. Even in the depths of winter, hard frosts made the ground a silvery winter wonderland, and magical mists turned my little world into a scene from *The Lord of the Rings* movies.

The Importance of Nature

If you look the right way, you can see that the whole world is a garden.
—Frances Hodgson Burnett, *The Secret Garden*

Severe illness can trap you inside for days on end. If you then include hospital stays and lengthy periods waiting in corridors for medical appointments, you can start to dislocate from the real world. When spending all my time on a sofa or in bed, what I missed most was the feel of light rain against my cold cheeks, having walked my dogs in all weather daily for years. Not sunshine, as you might expect, but gentle rain.

It reminded me of when I lived and worked in London, spending my days in hermetically sealed air-conditioned offices and my home, an apartment, albeit with a balcony overlooking the Thames River. I remembered becoming desperate to feel the grass under my feet once again, so I filled the balcony with pots and plants.

One of the problems of chronic pain and illness is a sense of alienation from your own body, which is understandable given what it has put you through. Even when the body begins to heal, it can be hard to trust it once again. Why would you since it has been unreliable for so long? One of the ways to reestablish a sense of equilibrium is to purposely and mindfully reground yourself in nature. Tim Beiske, MD, who works with Deepak Chopra, writes, "Enveloping ourselves in the rhythms and the forms of nature can be transformative and healing" (chopra.com).

Ayurveda, the ancient healing system of India, recognizes the healing benefits of nature and recommends finding time to connect with it on four sensory levels, namely sight, sound, touch, and smell. Activating and indulging the senses in this way allows for a totally immersive experience in the natural world and is best accompanied by a sense of curiosity and delight. It is an excellent extension of living mindfully. The role of the evocative sounds of nature in promoting relaxation is evidenced by the range of soundtracks available as backgrounds for guided meditations. Also, massage, aromatherapy, and reflexology practitioners usually introduce tracks with the sound of the waves or the rainforest to their treatments.

Luckily, I have the English countryside in all its green richness surrounding my house, and although hardly able to walk, I could view a wealth of wildlife—rabbits, squirrels, and the occasional deer—through my windows and from my doorstep. An existing interest in birds increased, fed by an abundance of resident song and field birds and birds of prey. Pheasants, partridge, and guinea fowl—some no doubt escapees from local shoots—paraded by as I rested, while industrious green and rarer black-and-white woodpeckers poked for ants on the stone paving.

At night, the owls would hoot in succession through the trees or spook the terrier by gliding up behind him on silent wings such that he would scoot into the house with his tail tucked firmly between his legs. Not much freaked the terrier, but the owls did. I would be taken on drives to view the countryside, and after months largely housebound or hospital-bound, it is amazing how astoundingly large a patch of sky can seem.

I recommend regular interaction with the natural world as an antidote to the physical and mental stress of lupus, as well as an extension of living positively in the moment.

Beneficial Rituals

When tea becomes ritual, it takes its place at the heart of our ability
to see greatness in small things … in small things that aspire to
nothing, yet know how to set a jewel of infinity in a single moment.
—Muriel Barbery, *The Elegance of the Hedgehog*

As you concentrate and practice mindfulness more, you will find yourself savoring the details of your life with greater relish. An extension of living in the moment is the idea of establishing beneficial rituals within your life. It acknowledges that human beings are creatures of habit and that some of these habits are heartwarming, life affirming, and deeply comforting. The Japanese have elevated drinking tea to a complex ceremony and this is an example of a simple practice that has grown to have huge cultural and meditative significance.

This can be replicated on a smaller scale: "Rituals are beneficial in the sense that they create higher levels of enjoyment in the experience," wrote Harvard Professor Michael Norton, and he and his colleague Francesco Gino found that while performing rituals, "you feel better … regardless of belief" (Nobel 2013). Also recorded are Professor Kathleen Vohs's findings after a series of experiments that "rituals seem to work because they increase your involvement with the experience" (Vohs 2018). As an extension of mindfulness, you can elevate small repeated daily habits, such as your morning beverage in your favorite mug, into mini-rituals that are savored and which then become more life enhancing.

Mindfulness has had its critics. Miguel Farias and Catherine Wikholm, who, having witnessed the explosion in its popularity over the last decade, wrote *The Buddha Pill* to warn against it being seen as a universal cure. Nicholas van Dam, Marieke van Vugt, and David Vigo advised in 2017 that "misinformation and poor methodology" could lead to practitioners being "misled and disappointed" about mindfulness (van Dam 2017).

So Dr. Ken A. Verni, PsyD, director at the New Jersey Center for Mindfulness, which is modelled on and linked to Kabat-Zinn's original Center for Mindfulness in Massachusetts, takes great pains to point out that their mindfulness program is "designed to complement traditional medical treatments and is beneficial when used in conjunction with the standard treatments for many medical conditions" (mindfulawarenessnj.com). This is indeed the way I have used it, creating an additional beneficial layer to the existing medicines and other holistic treatments. Far from any one element being a cure-all, it is my experience that a multidimensional approach to this complex condition has the greatest impact.

With the breath work as a foundation, I introduced cognitive behavioral and mindfulness systems into my life, which tackled the erratic nature of the disease and the daily reality of the extended healing process. I no longer felt useless and completely helpless. Wholehearted practice equipped me with a set of tools that became second nature and retrained my mind to be less negative and less concerned. Now I had systems to overcome panic attacks and bouts of intense anxiety when they surfaced unbidden and unwanted. Over time, this combination built a sense of equilibrium that had been distressing in its absence.

CHAPTER 10

Valuable Meditation and Visualization

Don't pass judgment just pay attention.
—Gabriel Shaw

It is helpful to your daily functionality and the overall healing process that you find a calm center and a way of rebalancing back to that center. Mini-flares and bad days in particular can impact you emotionally as well as physically.

Prior to training as a counsellor and psychotherapist, I studied guided meditation and visualization at the College of Psychic Studies in South Kensington in London. This knowledge developed further during my psychotherapeutic training. With the extra benefit of highly experienced supervision, I employed both techniques powerfully when counselling young people with severe physical disabilities and learning difficulties; and I also used them with my adult clients. Now my reading and research revealed that meditation was considered beneficial for complex illnesses and pain.

A study led by Dr. Madhav Goyal at Johns Hopkins University in 2014 researched 3,515 participants across forty-seven trials with various mental and physical illnesses, including depression, anxiety, cancer, and chronic pain. After eight weeks of meditation, they found firstly that there was no harm done and secondly that "meditation appeared to provide as much relief from anxiety and depression symptoms as ... antidepressants" (Goyal 2014).

It has been noted that new brain imaging techniques have allowed scientists to explore how the brain is influenced by certain activities, and in recent years, some have found evidence that the prefrontal region, responsible for cognition, is strengthened by meditation. This, in turn, regulates the area responsible for emotions, namely the amygdala. This alteration in brain activity is thought to "be associated with more positive self-representation, higher self-esteem, and higher acceptance of oneself" (McKay 2017). Scientists have concluded the following: "Research over the last two decades broadly supports the claim that mindfulness meditation … exerts beneficial effects on physical and mental health, and cognitive performance" (Tang 2015).

Buddhists practice daily mindfulness meditation, and monks pursue it as an essential part of their path to enlightenment and Nirvana. Their techniques have spread to the wider world and are now practiced by many non-Buddhists in their search for tranquility and insight. The archetypal image of a Buddhist monk sitting perfectly calm while mayhem swirls around typifies the serenity that this meditation practice seeks. "Do not dwell on the past, do not dream of the future, concentrate the mind on the present moment" (Buddha).

Mindfulness meditation is a development of the breath work and daily mindfulness techniques, and as I had already put these in place, this became my primary form of meditation. As Davidji describes: "In mindfulness meditation, we keep bringing our awareness to all the experiences of the present moment—thoughts, sounds, physical sensations, our breath … whatever comes … wherever our attention goes in the moment. We keep coming back to the present—not the past, not the future, but the present" (Davidji 2012).

I started meditating by sitting comfortably and keeping warm, as I did with breathing exercises. Then I closed my eyes, which stills the powerful visual sense and turns consciousness inward. I began by concentrating on the breath as before and then added a simple two-stage affirmation such as "Today I am healing" or "I love my muscles; my muscles are my friends," with the first part on the inhale and the second on the exhale. The affirmation helped me to still my thoughts and enabled a transition to pure mindfulness, where I stopped the affirmation and merely focused on everything in the moment. Detaching myself from the normal relentless feed of information and from the constant swirl of self-talk, I simply acknowledged any intrusive thoughts without judgment and let them pass by like clouds in the sky.

Starting with ten minutes, I gradually built up to twenty minutes about four to five times a week in a good week. The goal is daily.

I found that merely taking the time to quiet the mind, when not suffering intense pain and/or nausea, was enormously helpful in reaching even higher levels of mind-body calm. The immediate benefit is relaxation, which reduces the stress hormone cortisol in the body. Lower stress levels mean less tension in the muscles, which helps stiffness and pain. Then you reach a point when that perfect little space in time becomes a safe harbor that you want to experience regularly. Dialing down the stress for the specific period builds a feeling of mental peace that extends beyond the practice. It seems to protect you from stress throughout the day and steadily creates a wider sense of emotional stability. "Calm abiding is a heightened state of awareness when your body and your mind become especially flexible, receptive, and serviceable" (His Holiness the Dalai Lama).

There are multiple forms of meditation and books on the subject. There are also several ways of being tutored, such as joining classes. I found Davidji's guidance one of the most useful in understanding the benefits. Although he writes, "I honor all schools of meditation," he now concentrates on primordial sound meditation, which is where a mantra, specific to the date of your birth, is given along with personalized training. This training is available from him at www.davidji.com or any of the 1,500 Chopra centers worldwide (www.chopra.com).

Guided Meditation

> If you can accept that there is suffering now but
> that it will pass, you will also suffer less.
> —Patrizia Collard

For those who find quietening the mind difficult, guided meditations and visualizations can be helpful and, again, there are many sources available. They can also be integrated powerfully with an existing meditation practice. The guided meditations by Paul R. Scheele are extremely helpful. They are based on more than two decades of research and fieldwork and combine neuro-linguistic programming techniques with integrated left and right brain learning into a series of recordings. Topics such as anxiety-free, deep relaxation, overcoming overwhelm, and the self-esteem supercharger, each of approximately twenty minutes long, can all be purchased and sent or downloaded. They can be played regularly for four to five times a week for a month. A set of earphones is required, as different messages are played into the left and right ears. It is one of those situations where even though you may not understand how it works, the impact can be profoundly relaxing and reassuring, with benefits building over time with repeated use. As the days continue, stresses, strains, and obsessions seem to diminish in importance or even lift away entirely.

It all comes down to finding a form of meditation that resonates with you. You should feel free to try different approaches, and some may work for a while before you move onto another form. The overall aim is for you to explore the possibility of adding beneficial layers of calm, relaxation, and support.

Please find below a guided meditation that is tailored to meet the specific challenges of lupus. This meditation is an extension of the progressive muscle relaxation technique but is adjusted for lupus. Progressive muscle relaxation is sometimes just called Jacobson's PMR after it was perfected by Edmund Jacobson, MD, PhD, in the 1930s. His premise was that "mental calmness is a natural result of physical relaxation," and his method is to tense each muscle group for ten seconds at a time, then relax, working downward from the top or upward from the bottom of the body, the inherent idea being that you cannot be anxious and stressed at the same time as your muscles are relaxed: "An anxious mind cannot exist in a relaxed body" (Jacobson 1929 and 1934). So that mental calmness is a natural result of the physical relaxation once the muscle clench is let go. Ultimately, the technique is looking to break the tense muscle/stressed mind cycle or, at its most basic, the fight-or-flight response in the peripheral nervous system and the brain. The overall aims are a state of relaxation and feelings of calm.

When experimenting with different methods to see if they would help my painful and rigid muscles, I tried this system out, having noticed elements of it creeping in to other influential peoples' guided meditations. However, there is one big problem if you have lupus, which is that the muscles are already likely to be so tense and painful that tightening them further hurts and is basically a distraction, making it unsuitable for meditation. So for those with lupus, I have amended the system to allow you instead to focus on each muscle group, thereby harnessing the power of intention. Then relax each muscle group. Combined with breath control, I have found this to be a far more beneficial system.

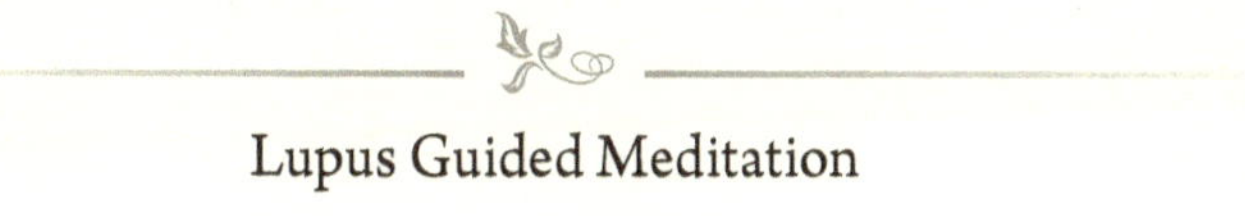

Lupus Guided Meditation

Close your eyes. Focus on the left foot, take a deep breath and let it out, relaxing the muscles in your left foot, and say aloud, "I acknowledge my pain, my deep, throbbing pain."

Breathe in and out. Focus on the right foot, take a deep breath and let it out, relaxing the muscles in you right foot, and say: "I acknowledge the relentless pain throughout my body."

Breathe in and out. Focus on the left knee, take a deep breath and let it out, relaxing the muscles all around your left knee, and say, "I acknowledge my fatigue, my sense of weakness."

Breathe in and out. Focus on the right knee, take a deep breath and let it out, relaxing the muscles all around your right knee, and say, "I acknowledge my deep, debilitating fatigue."

Breathe in and out. Focus on the left hip, take a deep breath and let it out, relaxing all the muscles around the left hip, and say, "I acknowledge my stress."

Breathe in and out. Focus on the right hip, take a deep breath and let it out, relaxing all the muscles around the right hip, and say, "I acknowledge my anxiety and stress, all my recurrent anxiety and stress."

Breathe in and out. Focus on the left hand, take a deep breath and let it out, relaxing all the muscles in your fingers, thumb, and wrist, and say louder, "I honor my determination through all this."

Breathe in and out. Focus on the right hand, take a deep breath and let it out, relaxing all the muscles in your fingers, thumb, and wrist, and say, "Through all this crazy stuff I have to deal with!"

Focus on the left shoulder, take a deep breath and let it out, relaxing all the muscles all around your shoulder, and say even louder, "I honor my bravery." Breathe in and out.

Focus on the right shoulder, take a deep breath and let it out, relaxing all the muscles around your right shoulder, and say, "My incredible courage in the face of all these symptoms, these truly awful symptoms."

Breathe in and out. Focus on your jaw, take a deep breath in and let it out, relaxing all the muscles in your jaw, right up into both ears, and say loudly, "Actually, I am amazing."

Breathe in and out. Focus on the crown of your head, take a deep breath in and out, relaxing all those small muscles covering the top of your head and down the back of your head, and reiterate, "I really am amazing!"

Breathe in and out and say with complete conviction, "I know for certain that I am surrounded by support and love and light." "In this moment and going forward." "By support and love and light, all around me."

Take a final deep breath in and out. Stretch gently and, when you are ready, open your eyes and assess how you feel now.

Again, you can use the record function on your phone to put this into your own voice and play it back. You can just stop at any point if you feel light-headed or uncomfortable and then just pick back up where you left off.

Positive Visualizations

> Positive thinking is powerful thinking.
> —Germany Kent

Positive visualization is one of the leading tools of modern sports psychology. It is based on the principle that where the mind leads, the body follows. Returning to golfing analogies, it is all too easy when standing on the tee, with a large hazard between you and the green, to think, *What I really don't want to do here is to hit the ball into the water. Yes, I absolutely must not hit the ball into the water—that would be dreadful.* Why is it that overturning the odds, nine times out of ten the ball flies straight into the hazard, leaving you saying, "But that was exactly what I did *not* want to do!"

Well, the wrong outcome happened because your body did not hear the word *not*, instead, it merely followed through with what you had pictured in your mind, which was the shot going wrong. Furthermore, as we explored earlier in self-talk, you fueled the wrong outcome with negative emotion: "The problem with most people is that they program their subconscious mind with negative coordinates. They visualize images of failure, they replay mistakes, they think about the negative scenarios that might happen, and picture the negative consequences that might arise" (Neason 2012).

Your subconscious cannot make a qualitative judgment, and you should not ask it to. So you need to remove the negative picture and the mental constructs and replace them instead with a crystal clear detailed image of what you want to happen. In this format, positive imagery becomes a natural extension of positive goal setting, as has been discussed in detail.

So for those with lupus, the way to harness this technique is to build a scenario, like a scene from a movie, of what you are doing when significantly improved or in remission. I created a mental video of me driving to my favorite store on my own (clearly not weak and not on heavy painkillers) and then parking, jumping down from my car, and walking freely into the store (not in a wheelchair). I imagined in detail what I was wearing and purchasing freely and easily (no pain, no shuffling, no bent fingers and hands).

Then you need to practice this, for five minutes a day or whenever you remember. It is important that your internal commentary does not futurize the picture, as in, "When I am better, I *will* do this," because this then places the scenario permanently out of reach. Rather, you must imagine it firmly in the present tense. This ability to think in real time will be enhanced by all your mindfulness practice, while your positive self-talk procedures will stand you in good stead for quelling any negative commentary that might seep in.

Personal experience and training, supported by wider reading on my tablet, gave me the ideas for these techniques. Then experimentation eliminated those psychological and behavioral methods which were not useful or which did not suit severe lupus. Repetition embedded these new norms of positive thinking and mindfulness. Meditation, guided meditation, and visualization added fresh layers of calm. I gained a new perspective that bad days were just that, bad days with physical and emotional symptoms that would pass. Despite the continued pain and erratic path of my medical condition, I became calmer, more content, and steadily more resilient.

PART III

HOLISTIC PHYSICAL SOLUTIONS

CHAPTER 11

Optimum Nutrition for Lupus

He that takes medicine and neglects diet wastes the skills of the physician.
—Chinese proverb

Given the complexities of testing, diagnosis, and medications, it is perhaps understandable that diet is often an afterthought for this condition. Nevertheless, in pursuing a multilayered method where no stone is left unturned, dismissing diet is unwise. In fact, the food you eat is a fundamental building block of this recommended holistic approach to lupus.

Weakness, extreme fatigue, digestive upset, pain, and nausea can all make eating properly with lupus enormously difficult, while corticosteroid cravings and mood swings further complicate matters. In my experience, pursuing a labor-intensive or ultra-strict eating regime can be nigh impossible. There are days, even weeks in some cases, such as mine, when producing and digesting a meal can be challenging. Dietary advice for lupus needs to be flexible in the face of this reality. It also needs to give direction about what will exacerbate symptoms and point to readily available sources of desperately needed high-quality nutrition.

Lupus Allergens

Given that systemic lupus erythematosus is known to generate sensitivities throughout the body, you will not be surprised to know that lupus patients are especially susceptible to dietary intolerances and allergic reactions. There are certain foods that are specifically contraindicated for lupus, and these are dealt with first.

Celiac disease is an autoimmune disorder, and as we have already identified, people with one autoimmune disease are prone to other autoimmune conditions. It is where the small intestine becomes inflamed because of an adverse reaction to a protein called gluten. Gluten is found in three types of cereal grains, namely wheat, rye, and barley, and in any foods containing these grains, including pasta, bread, cakes, biscuits, some sauces, and some ready meals. Leading symptoms of the disease are diarrhea, abdominal pain, bloating, gas, weight loss, and fatigue.

Clinical research has put the level of people with lupus and full-blown celiac disease at only 2 percent to 3 percent but acknowledged the following: "This study suggests that SLE occurs far more frequently in biopsy-defined coeliac [English spelling] disease than is currently appreciated" (Freeman 2008). Therefore, gluten intolerance, if not full-blown celiac disease, is thought to be more widespread.

The symptoms of irritable bowel syndrome (IBS) are pain and cramping, alternating constipation and diarrhea, gas and bloating. As we have already identified, lupus can adversely target the length of the alimentary tract, and this includes digestion. It can instigate celiac- or IBS-type symptoms, or it can heighten other typical symptoms such as fatigue and weakness, painful joints, and depression. During what I recognize with hindsight to have been a flare in the early 1990s, a blood test by my doctor diagnosed me as being intolerant to gluten, and I have followed a gluten-free diet ever since. Although now relatively common, it was rare at the time, and on the first trip to the supermarket following diagnosis, there seemed to be practically nothing gluten-free.

Nowadays, this is no longer the case, and both food stores and restaurants are far more accommodating. Nonetheless, it is important to recognize that some products merely replace gluten with higher levels of refined sugar and with high-glycemic starches, including potato and tapioca, which may be indigestible for those with sensitive stomachs. As Dr. Christiane Northrup notes, "The biggest problem with foods labelled 'gluten-free' is their reliance on highly processed ingredients such as cereal grains, soy, industrial seed oils, and sugar, which are low in nutrients and high in toxins."

Another allergy specifically identified with lupus is the so-called "nightshade" allergy, which refers to vegetables belonging to the Solanaceae family and which includes the following:

- Tomatoes and tomatillos
- Potatoes (but not yams and sweet potatoes)
- Eggplants (or aubergines)
- Peppers including bell peppers, chilies, tamales, pimentos, paprika, and cayenne pepper

Prepared foods that may contain nightshades include the following:

- Pickles and soups
- Mexican, Italian, and Indian foods
- Those using potato starch as a thickening agent
- Pizza
- Tomato sauce, salsas, ketchup, and red pepper seasonings
- Tobacco

Nightshade allergy symptoms often overlap with those of a gluten allergy in that they can include rashes, nausea, stomach bloating, anemia, headaches, joint pain, and low mood.

Other Contraindications for Lupus

Two other side effects of corticosteroid use are extra fluid retention and high blood pressure, and in both cases, a low-sodium diet is recommended. *Low* is different from *none,* with athletes understanding the importance of maintaining their bodies' electrolytes with salt.

Salt is a vital source of some crucial minerals such as iodine, which is needed by the body to ensure the proper functioning of the thyroid gland, which controls the body's metabolism. Thyroid problems, as previously discussed, can be comorbid with lupus.

Unfortunately, fine white table salt is superheated to make it refined and chemicals in the form of anticaking agents are added. Therefore, for those with lupus, small amounts of sea salt, which is generally lower in sodium than table salt and retains its beneficial minerals and trace elements, is a much better alternative. Connoisseur salts are a specialist area, but of these, pink Himalayan salt, which is harvested from historic seabeds in the relatively unpolluted Himalayas, is particularly rich in minerals that are thought to assist with muscle cramps. So you might wish to consider adding this to your kitchen cupboard of healthier condiments and seasonings.

A number of herbs taken as supplements and in teas are contraindicated with leading lupus medications. According to recent research published in the *British Journal of Clinical Pharmacology*, "clinically significant interactions" were found between patients taking warfarin and herbal medicines containing **St John's Wort**, for depression and low mood, and **cranberry**, for cystitis. The research concluded that these herbs might reduce the anticoagulant abilities of warfarin (Awortwe 2018).

Ginkgo biloba is one of the world's oldest living tree species, with some specimens living for over a thousand years, and is a very popular herbal supplement for treating memory problems and as an antioxidant. It is advised that it too can interfere with blood-thinning medications such as warfarin and aspirin. It is also contraindicated with antidepressants, selective serotonin reuptake inhibitors or SSRIs, where it can increase the risk of the potentially life-threatening serotonin syndrome. It is also contraindicated if you are on immunosuppressants, and it is thought to lessen the impact of the anxiety drug alprazolam. In summary, if you are on these medications it is best not to take ginkgo biloba without first consulting your doctor.

Alcohol is contraindicated, especially with opioid painkillers, which already cause drowsiness and narcoleptic tendencies.

Foods that Promote Inflammation in the Body

Aside from foods that are specifically detrimental and that may need to be eliminated from the lupus diet, there are also foods and categories of foods that, especially in large and regular quantities, exacerbate leading negative lupus symptoms, such as inflammation and low mood. These are as follows:

- Alfalfa
- Soy

- Processed fats and oils
- Highly processed, refined carbohydrates such as white flour
- Processed, refined white sugar

Alfalfa seeds and sprouts (but not the leaves) contain the amino acid L-canavanine, which can stimulate the immune system, triggering lupus-like symptoms, including muscle pain, fatigue, abnormal blood test results, and kidney problems.

Soy products are high in phytoestrogen, which is being researched as a potential risk factor for people with lupus. No direct causal link has yet been made between estrogens and soy isoflavones, but caution about including large amounts of soy in a lupus diet is advised.

Processed vegetable oils such as corn or palm oils are high in the inflammatory fat omega-6 and low in beneficial omega-3. When these oils are fried at high temperatures, they also produce something called advanced glycation end products, or AGEs. "Skin is the largest organ in the body," and research has shown that AGEs "decrease skin elasticity" and has concluded that "there is ample evidence that AGEs play an important role in skin aging" (Gkogkolou and Böhm 2012). The study goes on to note that, on the other hand, green tea and vitamins C and E specifically inhibit skin glycation. For people with lupus, it is recommended that **olive oil**, both light and extra virgin, is the most nutritious oil to use, with sunflower or canola oil used in moderation at higher temperatures.

Refined white flours are processed until a large proportion of the beneficial nutrients and fiber have been eliminated. Digestion can break down these foods rapidly, and this can spike insulin levels, which increases the inflammatory response in the body. In addition, many standard white flours contain pesticides, preservatives, and bleaching agents that increase the level of toxins in the system. Raising toxicity is just asking an out-of-balance system—already fighting a great deal—to take on more.

Foods that Beneficially Offset Drug Side Effects

People with lupus are routinely given corticosteroids, often in high doses, either orally or intravenously, especially at the onset of flares, as discussed. As history shows, the introduction of corticosteroid treatment has been groundbreaking and lifesaving, but one of the major problems with corticosteroids can be bone impairment.

Research in 2000 confirmed the following: "Clinically and statistically significant prevention of bone loss at the lumbar spine and forearm with vitamin D and Calcium in corticosteroid patients" (Homik 2000). Most foods are poor sources of vitamin D, and this vitamin is different from other foods in that our own bodies manufacture the majority of the required amount by exposure to sunlight. Due to the light sensitivity of those with lupus, they are specifically advised to avoid sunlight and to wear high factor SPFs or to cover up when going outside to prevent discoid rashes and systemic reactions, including fatigue and joint pain.

For this reason, "vitamin D plus calcium is superior to no therapy or calcium alone and should be given as a baseline therapy to prevent or treat steroid-induced osteoporosis" (Jehle 2003). Those with lupus are now routinely recommended to take daily calcium plus vitamin D supplements given the importance of preventing bone loss if corticosteroids are being taken. Indeed, the National Health Service in the UK usually gives it as a prescription. Despite supplements, it is also advised that people with lupus should make foods high in good-quality calcium and vitamin D part of their diet.

Foods High in Vitamin D

- Oily fish such as salmon
- Cheese
- Egg yolks
- Beef liver

Note that any kind of offal should be organic or from a trusted source because these organs process and store any antibiotics, hormones, and pesticides that are fed to nonorganic cattle, pigs, lamb, and poultry.

Foods High in Calcium

- Cheese
- Yogurt
- Seafood

- Sardines and salmon
- Beans and lentils
- Dried fruit
- Tofu
- Almonds
- Seeds including poppy, sesame, celery, and chia seeds

Many aged hard cheeses, while dense with calcium, are also lower in lactose, making them easier to digest. Similarly, goat and sheep cheeses contain a greater number of short- and medium-chain fatty acids than cow's milk, again making them easier for those with digestive weakness or a tendency to intolerances. When first diagnosed as being gluten intolerant in the early 1990s, it was recommended that I eat only goat and sheep's milk products instead of cow's milk products. These are easier to digest and kinder to an inflamed gut. Although I was able to gradually reintroduce cow's milk back into my diet, I still emphasize the use of goat and sheep's milk products, where possible, to decrease the burden on my system.

Yogurt is especially valuable because, along with being an easily digestible protein and providing calcium, it contains beneficial bacteria that aid digestion, such as bifidobacterium, lactobacillus bulgaricus, and streptococcus thermophilus. As explored previously, the alimentary tracts of people with lupus are often sources of numerous problems along their full length. This, combined with the side effects of drugs closely associated with lupus, and in particular pain relievers and antibiotics for infections, makes it especially important to eat natural yogurt regularly.

Nutrition to Offset Lupus Symptoms

Anemia is estimated to manifest in "about half of all people with active lupus" (Rosove 2013), with fatigue being one of the first and leading signs. The body must continuously replace red blood cells on an approximate 120-day cycle, and deficiency can be the result of inflammation, problems with hormone stimulation in the kidneys, iron deficiency, and bone marrow loss. The latter is sometimes a side effect of immunosuppressant drugs such as azathioprine and cyclophosphamide. It is usual for patients with lupus to have regular tests for blood and kidney health and to be prescribed a daily iron supplement to ensure against anemia. Maintaining good levels of iron in the diet is also recommended, and iron-rich foods include the following:

<u>Foods Rich in Iron</u>

- Red meat and chicken (grass-fed and organic meats will be richer in minerals and without ingested pesticides, growth hormones, and antibiotics).
- Eggs (again, organic eggs or free-range eggs from a trusted local source should be free from hormones, antibiotics, and ingested vaccines; and the yolks have been shown to be richer in vitamins A, E, beta-carotene, and omega-3 and lower in cholesterol than battery-farmed eggs).
- Fish, especially tuna and sardines.
- Tofu, lentils, and soybeans.
- Green leafy antioxidant-rich vegetables such as kale, spinach and Swiss chard.
- Pulses, beans, and wholegrains such as brown rice, quinoa, and oatmeal.
- Nuts, seeds, and dried fruit, including pumpkin.
- Blackstrap molasses and prune juice.

There are two types of iron, namely heme and nonheme. Heme iron is found in animal meat and is more easily absorbed; nonheme, which is plant-based, is somewhat less easily absorbed. Therefore, it is worth noting that vegetarians and vegans may have lower stores of iron than omnivores and may need to work that much harder to ensure no shortfall in their intake.

<u>Foods That Fight Inflammation</u>

As we have stated in earlier chapters, systemic inflammation is a hallmark of lupus, and Harvard Women's Health Watch noted in August 2017, "One of the best ways to quell inflammation lies not in the medicine cabinet but in the refrigerator." In keeping with this process of putting in place as many beneficial layers as possible in a holistic approach to lupus, eating foods that quell inflammation in the body makes good sense. Foods that specifically fight inflammation in the body are as follows:

- Green leafy vegetables such as kale, chard, bok choi, and lettuce
- Celery
- Nuts such as almonds and walnuts in their raw state or lightly cooked but not salted.
- Fatty fish such as salmon, mackerel, tuna, and sardines
- Wild meats such as duck and venison
- Grass-fed beef and lamb
- Olive oil
- Coconut oil
- Turmeric
- Ginger

Dark-colored fruits such as red apples, blueberries, cherries, strawberries, and raspberries contain powerful antioxidants and anti-inflammatories.

Orange and yellow fruits such as oranges, apricots, cantaloupe, melons, papayas, and mangos, in addition to vegetables such as carrots and sweet potatoes, all contain high levels of vitamin A, together with vitamin C, potassium, flavonoids, and lycopene. Vitamin A and lycopene are building blocks for the eyes and vision, while vitamin A on its own regulates the immune system and supports the function of the major organs, such as the lungs, kidneys, and heart, all of which can be harmed by lupus.

Ginger is especially beneficial for lupus and other autoimmune conditions because it "is an immune modulator that helps to reduce inflammation caused by an overactive immune response" (Dr. Axe). It is also an excellent digestive aid, alleviating nausea and heartburn.

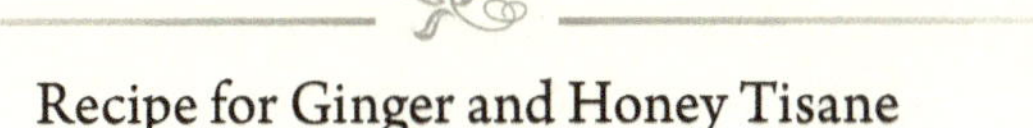

Recipe for Ginger and Honey Tisane

Approximately 10 grams peeled raw ginger, grated
1 teaspoon raw honey
Combine in a mug and add 1 1/2 cups of filtered water, boiled and then

cooled for two minutes to protect the beneficial properties of the raw honey. Stir.

<u>Potassium-Rich Foods</u>

Potassium-rich foods flush out toxins from the system, and key foods in this area are celery, beets, and broccoli. Potassium-rich sources include bone broth, which is also hugely beneficial because it is an easy-to-absorb method of obtaining the minerals chondroitin and glucosamine, compounds that are specifically helpful for arthritis symptoms and joint pain. Glucosamine is more suited to long-term joint deterioration and, as such, is better indicated for rheumatoid arthritis than lupus. You may recall from the earlier chapters that although responsible for pain and inflammation, lupus does not damage the joints in the same way as RA, but because it is in the same group of autoimmune conditions, people with lupus may also develop RA. Chondroitin sulfate functions by increasing water and lubrication around joints, thereby improving flexibility, and it helps the connective tissue that lines the gastrointestinal tract. One of the best ways to obtain and absorb glucosamine and chondroitin sulfate is via bone broth, although these minerals can also be taken in supplement form.

It is worth noting that if patients have advanced lupus nephritis, they are advised to follow a low-sodium diet. Chronic kidney disease can also lead to a condition called hyperkalemia, where failing kidneys no longer work efficiently to remove potassium from the body. In these rarer instances, patients are advised to follow a low-potassium diet.

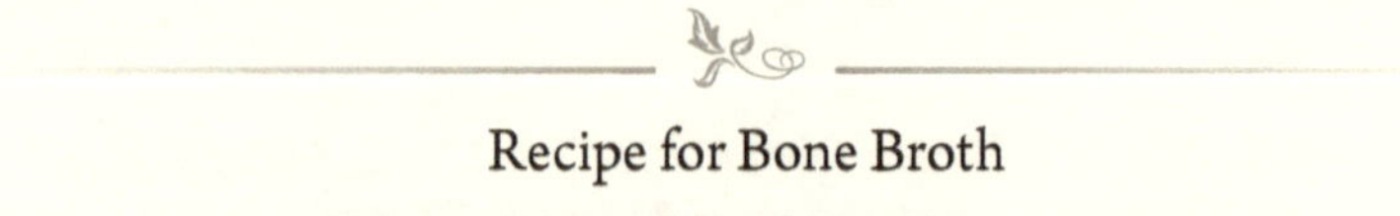

Recipe for Bone Broth

Carcass and bones of a roasted organic chicken or wild duck (other wild or organic poultry such as pheasant and lamb, as well as beef bones, are also acceptable, but it is critical not to use inorganic bones or carcasses, as these may have been exposed to antibiotics and growth hormones. The bones need to be cooked prior to use for broth).

150 grams celery, roughly chopped
150 grams carrots, roughly sliced
I medium onion, cut into quarters
½ teaspoon black peppercorns
3 bay leaves

Place in a large stewing pot with enough filtered water to cover the contents generously, bring to a boil, and simmer for three hours, partially covered, topping up with water as it evaporates.

Remove scum from the top and pass through a fine kitchen sieve or muslin. Pour into a jug and refrigerate, or put a portion into containers and freeze for future use.

It can be eaten with shredded cooked poultry, noodles, fresh coriander and spring onions, or used as a base for soups, risottos, and added to stir-fries.

Foods that are rich in **omega-3**, which cannot be produced by the body so a fresh supply must be gained from the diet, are highly beneficial and are to be found in fish, flaxseeds, nuts (especially walnuts), and green leafy vegetables. Omega-3 is especially important for a healthy heart and the avoidance of strokes.

The Role of Sweet Foods

Human beings have a natural predilection for sweet things, possibly because this may have given an evolutionary advantage in seeking out the ripest fruits or hunting down high-energy honey. It is recorded that the ancient peoples of the Kalahari Desert, the Bushmen, had a special place in their culture for the foraging and eating of wild honey.

At the end of the twentieth century, a pediatrician named Cabajal carried out a study of the impact of using sugar on babies undergoing painful procedures in his maternity ward and concluded that the sugar had an analgesic—in other words, a pain-relieving implication—for infants. He therefore recommended that glucose and fructose "should be widely used for minor procedures in neonates" (Carbajal 1999), and a further study in 2008 "showed that the Premature Infant Pain Profile was significantly lower among newborns who received sucrose" (Taddio 2008). So there may be an inbuilt tendency in humans, particularly those in pain, to seek out sweet things.

People with lupus who are often battling chronic pain may therefore crave sweetness in their diets as a comfort food. However, ultrarefined sucrose enters the bloodstream fast and creates a quick sugar rush and a spike in mood. Unfortunately, this is quickly followed by a rapid crash because it is not underpinned by any quality nutrients, and over time, this erratic cycle can actually harm mental health. "Sweet food has been found to induce positive feelings in the short term ... People experiencing low mood may eat sugary foods in the hope of alleviating negative feelings. Our study suggests that a high intake of sugary foods is more likely to have the opposite effect on mental health in the long term" (Knuppel 2017). Nevertheless, it is acknowledged that it is easy when fatigued and depressed, classic lupus symptoms, to reach for the quick fix of that white sugar rush.

White sugar has been refined to the point where it contains no beneficial nutrients, which is why it is known as "empty calories." It enters the body via the digestive tract, where it is broken down into glucose and fructose. Corn syrup is another highly refined form of sucrose widely used in manufactured food products because it is cheaper but also some 20 percent sweeter than white sugar. Small amounts of fructose can easily be handled by the liver—for example, an amount contained in a piece of fruit—but in large amounts, it is not fully processed and is stored instead as fat (fat, of course, can also be a problem for those on corticosteroids). Too much sucrose is also linked to insulin spikes and eventually to resistance and type 2 diabetes; elevated blood pressure and liver disease; and to increased inflammation in the body, leading to cardiovascular disease, arthritis, and gout.

For people whose systems are already imbalanced and under stress and for whom inflammation is harmful, it is vital to avoid refined white sugar and refined fructose. Weight gain as a side effect of corticosteroids may already present a problem, and these refined sugars are bad for your dental and oral health too, as harmful bacteria in the mouth and throat easily use them. As we have stated earlier, lupus can pose additional dental, oral, and esophageal difficulties.

Instead, you should replace these cravings with moderate amounts of higher-quality alternatives. **Unrefined cane sugar** is derived from sugarcane, and the top five countries in the world in which it is grown are Brazil, India,

China, Thailand, and Pakistan, where its by-products are sustainably used as animal feed. Unrefined cane sugar, while more expensive than its white counterpart, contains a range of beneficial nutrients and minerals, including iron, magnesium, potassium, phosphorus, and calcium, and it also lacks the harmful substances that can be added to pure white sugar, such as sulfur dioxide.

Sulfur dioxide is a particular problem with white sugar manufactured in India, where it is used in the crystallization and the bleaching stages, known as "the double sulphitation process." Unfortunately, in this specific process, trace amounts of sulfur dioxide are left behind and are then responsible for respiratory problems, and this is why Indian white sugar cannot be exported to markets in the United States and Europe. Nevertheless, India is the world's second-largest producer of sugar behind Brazil, which dominates the market. Lower in calories than white sugar, unrefined cane sugar releases more slowly into the bloodstream and if consumed, again in moderation, can be used as a weight-for-weight alternative to white sugar for baking and cooking.

Dried fruits such as apples, dates, figs, apricots, and papaya also offer alternatives. With the majority of their water extracted, these become condensed easy-to-eat packages of vitamins and minerals. Furthermore, if they are combined with nuts for protein, they provide a far better answer for sweet cravings than processed chocolate bars and biscuits, especially for those with chronic health conditions.

There are sweet foods that are particularly beneficial because they offer both anti-inflammatory and antibacterial properties, and the two standout foods in this category are raw, unrefined honey and pineapple.

Raw honey, which is unfiltered and unpasteurized, is a superfood, as it contains both bee pollen (a ball of field-gathered flower pollen) and bee propolis (used as a sealant for open spaces in the hive), and it is a powerhouse of antiviral, antibacterial, and antifungal properties. It is also rich in vitamins and minerals that can reduce inflammation, including Vitamins A, E, and D and minerals such as calcium, iron, potassium, and selenium.

A 2010 study revealed that honeybee pollen mix displayed meaningful anti-inflammatory properties when given to mice with liver problems: "Honeybee pollen mix displayed significant … anti-inflammatory activities [at high doses taken orally] without inducing any apparent acute toxicity or gastric damage" (Kuppeli Akkol 2010).

A biological study of the benefits of different types of raw Thai honey in 2015 proved antibacterial and anti-inflammatory properties and concluded, "Honey demonstrates tremendous potential as a useful source that provides anti-free radicals, anti-tyrosinase, and antibacterial activity against pathogenic bacteria" (Jantakee and Tragoolpua 2015). Tyrosinase, an oxidizing enzyme found in plant and animal tissues, causes blackening of those tissues, hence the ability of honey to inhibit the blackening of wounds.

A teaspoon of raw honey can be eaten to benefit sore throats, spread on good-quality bread or rice cakes, added to dressings for salads, or used in hot drinks. If adding to hot drinks then you should wait two minutes before pouring over the water after boiling, as too high of a heat can destroy the beneficial enzymes and microbes, as has already been advised.

Pineapple, loved for its sweetness and juiciness, has substantial amounts of vitamin C. Drinking just one cup of juice or eating a one hundred gram portion will provide over 50 percent of your recommended daily intake of vitamin C. Pineapple is also special because it alone amongst fruits contains bromelain, an enzyme that helps digest protein and aids the colon. It should be noted that for a few people, pineapple can have the opposite result and irritate the stomach lining.

In 2014, a study into the impact of pineapple on dental bacteria found that: "Bromelain exerts an antibacterial effect against potent periodontal pathogens: hence it may be used as an antibacterial agent" (Praveen 2014). Although it is recognized that further research into the benefits is needed, pineapple is a good choice for people with lupus. It has anti-inflammatory, anti-free radical, and antibacterial properties, the latter being especially beneficial for those suffering with mouth ulcers and on immunosuppressant drugs. If it can be tolerated well, then pineapple is also good for joints.

Natural Mood-Enhancing Foods

While white sugar triggers a short-lived improvement in mood, other foods can improve mood more sustainably. **Tryptophan** is key to making serotonin, and without it, serotonin will not be produced because the body cannot make its own tryptophan. So it must be absorbed via the diet or as a supplement. After eating tryptophan, the body converts it into serotonin, melatonin, and vitamin B6. Serotonin helps to regulate mood, and it is sometimes called the happiness chemical, with low levels linked to depression (McIntosh 2018). Good sources of the essential amino acid tryptophan are often in high-protein foods such as eggs, cheese, red meat, tofu, salmon, beans, lentils, nuts, and turkey. Tryptophan also occurs naturally in high amounts in the following fruits and vegetables: pineapple, bananas and plantains, seaweed, spinach, watercress, broccoli, and bamboo shoots.

Dark chocolate with high concentrations of cocoa, at 70 percent, has been shown in recent studies, when eaten in moderation, to positively benefit brain function, improving stress levels, mood, and memory, according to a recent study published in April 2018.

The Importance of a Balanced Diet

Judith Wurtman, PhD, former director of the Women's Health Program at the Massachusetts Institute of Technology (MIT) and co-founder of the Adara Weight Loss Center, also in Boston, researched the connection between mood and **low-carbohydrate diets.** She discussed her findings with Brenda Goodman, who reported them in *Psychology Today* in 2016. Wurtman found that rats placed on a low-carb diet for three weeks had lower levels of serotonin. This study supported her own anecdotal evidence and observations from her positions at MIT and Adara: low-carbohydrate diets have a tendency to promote depression.

Despite the media popularity of low-carb diets such as Atkins and other ketogenic eating programs, in Wurtman's experience, they can present mental health problems. Despite the difficulties that corticosteroids can present with weight, her work suggests that extended low-carb eating is not suitable for those patients battling with the wider psychological implications of lupus. It is for this reason that a well-balanced diet incorporating high-quality slow-release carbohydrates is recommended instead. Sources of such carbohydrates would be organic or locally grown potatoes (if you do not have a nightshade allergy); sweet potatoes (exempt from nightshade allergy); brown rice and specialty rice like Arborio and basmati; oat, spelt and rye flours; corn; beans; and pulses.

It is also essential that a lupus diet is rich in **protein,** with a minimum requirement of eighty grams per day, especially if you have moderate or severe lupus and/or are experiencing regular flares or are recovering from a major flare. To meet basic dietary requirements, the recommended amount of protein is fifty-six grams per day for a man and forty-six grams of protein a day for a woman, but this alters if the person is very active or is recovering from ill health. When first identified as being allergic to gluten in the early 1990s, and because I was very weak and run down because of (with hindsight) a flare, I was advised by my doctor to eat a high-protein diet to help me recover, with a minimum of eighty grams of excellent-quality protein per day. Sources of such protein include organic or local farm poultry, fish, grass-fed beef and lamb, venison, organic or high-quality free-range eggs, cheese, and unsalted nuts and seeds, especially almonds.

Maximizing Nutrients

Juicing is a way of packing high-quality ultra-fresh ingredients into the body for maximum nutritional benefits with good digestibility. A greater quantity of fruits and vegetables can be condensed into a glass and drunk than can be eaten in one sitting, and they can be an important addition to a lupus diet, especially if you are looking to build yourself up between flares or are suffering from dysphagia (experiencing difficulty swallowing).

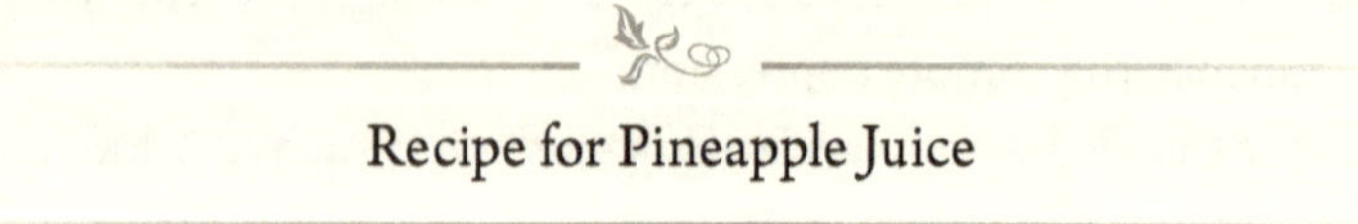

Recipe for Pineapple Juice

Half a medium-sized pineapple, peeled, de-eyed, and cored
2 green apples, washed but not peeled
35 grams ginger (or to taste), peeled

Hydration

With feverishness and nausea both common lupus symptoms, adequate hydration is of increased importance. In my own experience, you are more likely to be thirsty with lupus. Medications such as laxatives can further dehydrate the body. Drinking higher levels of water will aid with the production of saliva if you have Sjögren's syndrome, lubrication around joints, and the transit of waste through the bowels, as well as regulating body temperature during bouts of fever. A minimum of two liters of water per day for an adult is recommended just to prevent dehydration, without the additional requirements imposed by lupus symptoms and medication, so I follow an increase of 25 percent, for a minimum of 2.5 liters, including teas and juices. Mineral water also provides additional trace elements such as calcium, potassium, and magnesium.

In summary, the optimum lupus diet fulfils the following criteria:

- Avoids allergic foods such as nightshades and gluten
- Avoids foods that promote inflammation in the body
- Avoids processed and refined foods, especially white sugar and fine white salt
- Avoids foods high in toxins such as pesticides and hormones
- Concentrates on foods high in nutrients, such as fresh, organic, free-range, or locally grown
- Follows a balanced approach that includes high-quality animal or vegetable proteins, fats, and carbohydrates
- Provides higher levels of hydration

Supplements for Lupus

It is recommended that in addition to a high-quality balanced diet, some supplements are taken to protect and enhance certain areas and functions of the body that are specifically negatively influenced by lupus and the medications associated with its treatment. All supplements and their amounts must be communicated to your doctor or consultant to ensure that he has all the information pertaining to your care and to ward against contraindications with prescribed orthodox medicines.

Vitamin A is important for the health of the eyes. It has been noted that even without the presence of Sjögren's syndrome, which leads to dry eyes, hydroxychloroquine is contraindicated with eye health, so additional support for the eyes is recommended. The recommended daily amount (RDA) is 900 IUs, with a tolerable upper limit of 3,000 IUs for adults.

A lack of **B vitamins** can contribute to tiredness and anemia, to swollen and cracked lips, and to swelling in the mouth and throat. B vitamins also aid energy and the nervous system, with a calming effect on the emotions. Although a good-quality diet should provide the majority of the B vitamins required, it is acknowledged that those with chronic health conditions and especially celiac disease or who are over fifty years old may need a supplement. A balance of B vitamins is important, which is why a complex daily formula is the easiest option, although of course pregnant women will also be advised to take additional **folic acid**.

Biotin is a water-soluble B vitamin that is also referred to as B7 and is often taken specifically to improve the health of skin, hair, and nails. It is also thought to benefit mucus membranes and nerves. The RDA for biotin is 300 milligrams per day, but it is normal for supplements specifically supporting hair and nail health to contain 600 milligrams.

While pineapple flesh and juice contain beneficial amounts of the anti-inflammatory enzyme **bromelain** (with evidence to suggest that it fights pain and swelling in the joints, although more research is required), a large amount is stored in the stem, which is not eaten. So for those suffering from acute inflammatory conditions such as lupus, a supplement may be helpful. There is no RDA for bromelain, but a dose of 1,500 milligrams is thought to be beneficial.

Vitamin C is an excellent source of antioxidants, and vitamin C protects cells and functions throughout the body, enhancing the performance of other supplements. In particular, it increases the ability to absorb iron. The Mayo Clinic advises that the RDA "for vitamin C is 65 milligrams to 90 milligrams per day, and the upper limit is 2,000 milligrams per day" (Zeratsky 2018). I take a minimum of 500 milligrams per day in supplement form.

Calcium and Vitamin D: As stated earlier, calcium is better absorbed if it is taken along with vitamin D. The recommended daily amount (RDA) of calcium for those on corticosteroids is between 600 and 1,200 milligrams depending on your level of corticosteroids, both current and historic, and on the status of your DEXA bone density scans. In the UK, these vitamins are prescribed as standard for those on corticosteroids in order to prevent bone damage.

Although 400 IUS to 800 IUS a day is the standard RDA of vitamin D, some studies suggest that a higher intake of 1,000 IUS to 4,000 IUS is needed to maintain optimal blood levels. My London diagnostician recommended that I take 2,000 IUS per day of vitamin D, and my blood tests confirm that despite staying out of the sun due to my lupus, I have consistently good levels of vitamin D.

Cod liver oil is one of the best sources of omega-3, at approximately 20 percent, and helps the pain and inflammation of joints and muscles. It also contains vitamins D and A. The standard dose is 1,000 milligrams per day.

Vitamin E nourishes the skin and the eyes and strengthens the body's natural defenses against infection. Although a clinical deficiency is rare and it is present in high-quality plant oils, nuts, wheat germ, cereals, and cereal products such as organic wholemeal bread, a supplement, given the problems with lupus patients' skin, is recommended. I take 800 IUS per day in the morning. Vitamin E can also be applied topically to help heal discoid scars.

We have already stated above that to avoid the danger of anemia, lupus patients are often prescribed an **iron** supplement as standard—for example, 210 milligrams per day of ferrous fumarate.

Magnesium is needed to ensure a strong bone structure and prevent osteoporosis. It is contained in foods rich in fiber, such as whole grains, green leafy vegetables, broccoli, and seeds and nuts, especially almonds. It is good for acid indigestion and has a laxative result so it addresses many lupus-related problems. Women in particular are often found to be deficient in magnesium. A daily supplement of 400 milligrams per day is recommended. Further on, you will see ahead that some can also be obtained via bath salts.

A high-quality daily **probiotic,** to protect against the detrimental impact of medications on the gut and to support the working of the gastrointestinal tract, is essential. Courses of antibiotics will destroy the beneficial bacterial lining in particular and, along with corticosteroids and immunosuppressants, can leave those with lupus susceptible to candidiasis. Painkillers, especially combined with iron supplements, will slow down the colon. Natural yogurt, as we have said previously, will provide beneficial bacteria, as will artisan cheese, but this will almost certainly need topping up with a daily probiotic supplement.

Turmeric contains curcumin, which gives curry its yellow color, and it has a long history of use in Ayurvedic medicine as a treatment for inflammatory conditions. "Research has shown curcumin to be a highly pleiotropic [producing or having multiple effects from a single gene] molecule capable of interacting with numerous molecular targets involved in inflammation" (Jurenka 2009). Its efficacy is enhanced if combined with black pepper, which increases its performance by some 2,000 percent (Shoba 1998). However, it is poorly absorbed by the bloodstream, so a supplement to boost intake is necessary to maximize benefits. Supplements can come in tablet form but also as a powder that can be added to soups, juices, and smoothies. Then freshly ground **black pepper** can be added to the diet as a standard seasoning along with low amounts of sea or specialty salt, as previously discussed.

The approach of this book is first to remove allergens and toxins, then to identify those foods that are of the greatest help to people with lupus and to demonstrate why. The aim is to layer beneficial options for both the body and the mind, with no single factor a miracle cure but instead each contributing something else positive: an ultimate sandwich, so to speak, of foods, beverages, vitamins, minerals, and trace elements.

This diet enabled me to rebuild my weight to within six pounds of my pre-flare condition, despite regular nausea and weakness. In conjunction with medication, my liver repaired dramatically to a safe condition, and my inflammation, although still susceptible to setbacks, steadily reduced. My hair, with the support of topical tonics, also regrew to its preinfection strength and abundance.

My study of the best nutrition for lupus is not exhaustive, and when my weight dropped to just over six stones, or eighty-four pounds, qualified nutritionists and dieticians were assigned to help me, and I would urge you to seek further professional advice if you are concerned about excessive weight loss or gain, allergies, or appropriate supplements.

I hope that you will now feel more confident about what to avoid and what to emphasize in your diet and will be able to relish those wonderful, beneficial foods especially suited to lupus, safe in the knowledge that you are adding another positive pillar to your overall physical and mental progress.

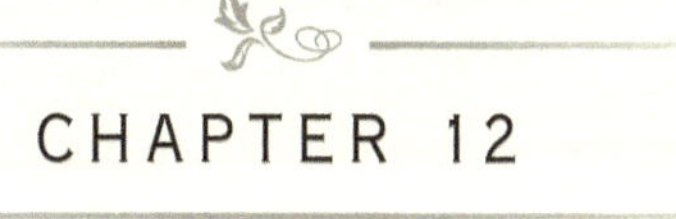

CHAPTER 12

Beneficial Body Work

Often the hands will solve a mystery that the
intellect has struggled with in vain.
—Carl Gustav Jung

The first pillar of this holistic approach to chronic pain and the other endemic symptoms of lupus is medical, the second is psychological, and the third is physical. By physical, I mean advice on the optimum diet, which has just been discussed, combined with complementary physical interventions and therapies that are particularly suited to this condition.

Heat

Think with the whole body.
—Taisen Deshimaru

If you have lupus, heat can be your friend. This is true of both climatic heat, with some patients having to actually move to warmer areas of the country to improve their symptoms, and applied heat. In my experience, cryotherapy products (freezing sensations) simply do not work as well as hot water bottles, heat pads, and heated blankets on sore and aching muscles or on localized areas of acute pain. The traditional link between swelling and ice is apparently more applicable to recent injury and treatment in the

145

first forty-eight hours of a sprain, for example, in conjunction with rest, compression, and elevation.

When combined with orthodox pain medications, heat can prove especially beneficial. The pain relief can either be taken orally, which is the standard approach, or ibuprofen gel can be massaged into painful joints and heat then applied on top with hot water bottles and heat pads.

Arnica is extracted from a European flowering plant called arnica montana, a member of the sunflower family noted for its yellow flower heads. It is used in herbal remedies and in homeopathy to help with swelling, inflammation, bruising, soreness, and aches and pains. It can come in the form of tablets, gels for topical application, massage oils, and crystals and oils for the bath. In all cases, look for pure extracts and products without mineral oils, synthetic fragrances or colors, parabens, silicates, or phthalates because lupus skin is highly sensitive, as we have previously stated. The gel can be massaged into the joint, just as with ibuprofen. Heat can then be applied on top, again in the form of hot water bottles or pads.

For some with lupus, muscle weakness and the sheer pain of getting into a bath, lying on a hard surface, and then pushing back out can make bathing impossible, so they have to shower instead. However, where symptoms do not prevent the pleasure of a hot bath, the following additions can directly help inflamed muscles and joints:

- **Arnica salts and oils** are often combined with juniper, ginger, and lavender for additional benefits.
- **Epsom salts** are a magnesium sulfate compound that can be dissolved in water, allowing these beneficial minerals to be absorbed through the skin (it can also be ingested, dissolved in water as a drink, and is a traditional remedy to alleviate constipation). The dissolved salts help to ease tired and aching muscles, relax the nervous system, and detoxify the body. It is beneficial for skin conditions such as psoriasis and eczema, but I can find no official recommendation for its use for cutaneous lupus or much anecdotal evidence for its use in this regard either. If you have a heart condition, high blood pressure, or diabetes, then you should consult with your doctor before taking Epsom salt baths.

- **Magnesium salts or flakes** are another form of magnesium, but this time magnesium chloride (unlike Epsom salts, they cannot be safely dissolved in water and ingested, although magnesium can also be taken in supplement form). Dissolved in a bath, they can help with aching muscles and joints, provide stress relief and relaxation, and again are soothing for the skin. There is some evidence that those who are chronically stressed tend to have reduced levels of magnesium in their systems, and magnesium deficiency can trigger higher levels of inflammation in the body. Therefore, there is a case for increasing your magnesium intake. This has been explored in the section on supplements, but clearly absorption through the skin may also be beneficial.

Whether you have Raynaud's or not, in my experience, keeping your extremities warm—fingers, hands, feet, and toes—is advantageous. Chinese medicine also recommends that it is important for the chronically ill to keep their cores cossetted with traditional kidney warmers. Personally, keeping my neck warm has also always proved important to ward against neck and shoulder pain. Fingerless gloves and wrist warmers are excellent for keeping vulnerable thumb and wrist joints comforted, even when in the house during winter, and can help with swelling and pain.

Massage

> We need four hugs a day for survival. We need eight hugs a day
> for maintenance. We need twelve hugs a day for growth.
> —Virginia Satir

Touch has been shown to be essential to psychological, emotional, and physical growth in infants, with numerous studies showing that a lack of touch results in underdevelopment. This is given the umbrella term "failure to thrive." "As recently as the 1990s, young children in Romanian orphanages were found to be physically undersized and emotionally unresponsive after lives deprived of sensory stimulation, especially touch" (Bruce 2015).

Lupus symptoms feed on stress. Endorphins are neuropeptides produced by the central nervous system and the pituitary gland. The pituitary gland is located in the brain just behind the nose, between the hypothalamus and the pineal gland, and is about the size of a pea. Endorphins release positive feelings in the body, and these feelings are described as euphoric, similar to the impact of opiates such as morphine on the central nervous system. This means that the body is capable of producing its own painkillers.

It is known that laughter and exercise instigate the release of endorphins, but relaxing body work has also been identified as a trigger. This book has covered the beneficial results of laughter, but as it concentrates on recovery from a bedridden and wheelchair-bound state, it does not address exercise in any detail beyond attaining basic daily functionality without pain. One of my goals is to incorporate gentle exercise when able, such as qigong, which is closely related to tai chi. "Qigong can be described as a mind-body-spirit practice that improves one's mental and physical health by integrating posture, movement breathing technique, self-massage, sound, and focused intent" (National Qigong Association). I also know that some with lupus find gentle yoga helpful. These forms of exercise work with the breath and do not tend to force the muscles or the joints. As such, they fit well with the gentle, holistic approach recommended in this book.

Returning to massage, it has been shown to reduce the stress hormone cortisol and, as well as endorphins, to release three other feel-good hormones, namely serotonin, oxytocin, and dopamine.

The ability of massage to provide healing touch and beneficial relaxation is subject to two caveats: Firstly, it is essential that you have an experienced masseuse who understands the body well and is capable of administering gentle but beneficial massages that do not instigate muscle or joint pain. They need to understand how to treat swollen and inflamed joints. It is the case for all complementary treatments that overly vigorous manipulation of the connective tissues (or joints) can definitely set off pain, mini-flares, and relapses; there is a great deal of anecdotal evidence on the lupus message boards to reinforce this.

Experience of treating patients suffering from chronic or severe illnesses can be worth checking for. My masseuse Ashley is a member of The Complementary Medicine Association in the UK. She is also a qualified radiographer with a degree in therapeutic radiography, and she set up her own mobile massage business to fit in with her growing children. She is able to untangle and soothe my rigid, painful muscles gently and skillfully, while inducing deep relaxation throughout my body. Most importantly, her treatments do not instigate pain, whether at the time or some hours later.

Secondly, again because of skin sensitivity, pure oils need to be utilized; indeed, you may want to supply your own tried-and-tested supplies. Safe aromatherapy oils for lupus are examined next.

My research has shown that Indian head massage and hot stone massage can also be beneficial for lupus.

I am still taking a medication called baclofen, which is usually for the effects of multiple sclerosis, spinal cord damage, and motor neurone disease. It was prescribed for me for when whole groups of my muscles went into spasm. You may recall that I described myself as feeling like the Tin Man from *The Wizard of Oz*. Regular massage has proved excellent at softening and relaxing my stiff and inflexible muscles.

Aromatherapy

> Aromatherapy is a truly holistic therapy, taking account of
> the mind, body, and spirit of the person seeking help.
> —Patricia Davis

Hypersensitivity seems to go hand in hand with physical fragility, including touch, taste, and smell. Therefore, it makes sense to harness an aspect of this vulnerability by incorporating essential oils.

Aromatherapy oils have both physical and emotional benefits. Applying the oils through massage has the physical advantages of relaxing the muscles and stimulating the circulation, while the smell of the oils triggers positive neurochemicals in the brain and improves negative emotions such as stress and depression.

The olfactory nerve in the nose is directly connected to the limbic system of the brain, which is responsible for moods and memories. This is why particular scents can be so evocative of a particular memory, such as your mother's baking or the smell of the sea from a childhood holiday. When you catch that scent again, it will take you back not only to the place but also to how you felt in that moment.

Research shows that the feel-good hormone oxytocin is stimulated by scenting certain smells, as well as by touch. Dr. Ray Sahelian's research into oxytocin discovered that it can have wider healing properties than previously thought and that it can "relax and reduce blood pressure and cortisol levels [and] has antianxiety effects." Calling it the "cuddle" hormone, he concluded that it "promotes growth and healing" (Sahelian 2010).

Those in chronic pain are often suffering from prolonged stress. The body releases cortisol in response to stress. In an emergency, this provides the body with glucose and the energy to fuel the fight-or-flight response so that you can run away extra fast from danger and have the clarity of mind to plan the best direction in which to run. However, if overstimulated by too much stress over too long a period, cortisol leads to increased blood sugar levels. This can lead to negative moods such as anxiety and depression, as well as weight gain.

One study found that increased stress and heightened cortisol levels reduced healing in healthy adult males, "indicating a clear elevation in the morning cortisol slope of those whose wounds were slowest to heal" (Elbrecht 2003). When working correctly, cortisol regulates the immune system. So it makes perfect sense to keep cortisol in balance when you are suffering from an autoimmune condition such as lupus.

For these collective reasons, essential oils should not be dismissed as just some nice smells but rather that aromatherapy can be part of the holistic tool kit for improving the quality of life for those with chronic pain and other debilitating lupus symptoms.

It is necessary to appreciate that essential oils are highly concentrated and too much can have adverse results, and they should only ever be applied externally. Furthermore, the tolerances of a well body are higher than those for someone with a chronic illness. Therefore, as a rule of thumb for those with lupus, both in terms of dilution strength and in the selection of the essential oils, it is safest to follow the advice for vulnerable categories of patients, namely those children over five years old, the elderly, and pregnant women. However, expert advice should be taken on the use of any aromatherapy oils in the first three months of pregnancy and throughout if there is a history of miscarriage. The leading child-, elderly- and pregnancy-safe oils are "lavender, frankincense, cedar wood, sweet orange, and roman chamomile" (Butje 2017).

Given their photosensitivity, lupus patients are advised to avoid those oils that also have this property. These are the citrus oils: lemon, lime (cold-pressed, not distilled, because it is phytotoxic in cold-pressed form but not in its distilled form), and sweet orange. Despite the fact that it scores on other measures of safety, sweet orange in direct contact with the skin is not suitable for lupus patients, but it can still be used in inhalers and diffusers.

Lavender is probably the best all-round essential oil and one of the safest. One of its main components is linalool, which research has shown to have profound benefits for the nervous system. Lavender is especially useful to lupus patients for its deeply relaxing and sleep-promoting properties, which can offset the tension and anxiety associated with the condition and the sleep disruption possible with corticosteroids. Many pillow sprays are available to aid sleep.

Frankincense: "One of my top picks for people with delicate systems" (Butje 2017). A leading oil for the improvement of skin, including scarring, frankincense has also long been associated with religious ceremony and is used in church services as an uplifting, spiritual scent. It is now often used as meditation oil. This has been one of my favorites through my lupus journey, and I often use it while meditating. It is, of course, heavily associated with Christmas, combined with pine and sweet orange. Myrrh has similar uses to frankincense, but according to Robert Tisserand and Rodney Young's book *Essential Oil Safety*, it is contraindicated for pregnancy, so I do not recommend here.

Cedar wood is another safe oil. Its woody scent is emotionally reassuring, and it calms the respiratory and nervous systems. For those suffering lung and breathing complications, it is highly recommended. It is famous for its insect repellent properties and is traditionally used in clothes and fabric storage to ward off moths.

Roman chamomile is used specifically for pain in the muscles and joints, and this is a calming and soothing oil that is good for alleviating stress.

Other oils that can have specific benefits for the symptoms of lupus include the following:

Palmerosa is good for warm and swollen joints and for emotional stress; it is a comforting oil.

Geranium is recommended for swollen joints, especially in the ankles and legs, for irritated skin, and is relaxing and an antidepressant.

German chamomile is good for inflammation in the muscles and joints, for pain relief and irritated skin, and is emotionally soothing. However, in *Essential Oil Safety*, by Robert Tisserand and Rodney Young, they point out that German chamomile may be contraindicated with some antidepressants and with the painkiller codeine (as well as the cancer drug tamoxifen).

Rosemary is recommended for joint pain and inflammation but also particularly for mental clarity. So it is good for lupus fog and can be sniffed from an inhaler to help keep a clear head.

As discussed, disruptions to the alimentary tract in general and the stomach specifically are common in lupus, and **peppermint** and **bergamot** are both excellent digestive oils. Unfortunately, peppermint can irritate the skin and eyes if applied topically or drops added to a bath; therefore, for lupus, it is best taken as an herbal tea. I have found it useful in this form for mild nausea. Bergamot, of course, is the famous ingredient in the traditional English beverage Earl Grey tea, with its relaxing and calming reputation.

Rose has a calming impact on the nervous system, but it can also be a heavy and cloying scent if too much is used, so for super sensitives, a single drop is recommended. However, it is a deeply nurturing oil and especially "loving" during difficult times.

Aromatherapy treatment comes with similar caveats to massage. Firstly, given the skin sensitivity and allergic bias of those with lupus, it is enormously valuable to ensure that the oils themselves are pure and additive-free, and the same rule applies to the carrier oils, gels, and waxes. Some experts emphasize the need to source organically grown and/or artisan-produced oils to maximize their benefits and to minimize possible negative reactions.

Secondly, aromatherapy massage should be inherently gentle, but it is best to seek out a qualified and experienced practitioner. Andrea Butje founded the Aromahead Institute in the United State, and it trains clinical aromatherapists. The Aromatherapy Council is a leading body for setting the standards for professional practice in the UK, and its fully trained aromatherapists blend oils especially to suit individual needs, doing so following a detailed consultation and in full knowledge of all relevant safety issues.

Reflexology

I see clients in "anxiety state" very often. This means that most
of their energy is in the head and the rest of the body is lacking in
enough energy to function well. Reflexology is thought to trigger
the parasympathetic nervous system, reducing anxiety, stopping the
"fight-or-flight" response, and allowing the body to heal itself.
—Rosanna Bickerton

Reflexology is based on the theory that areas and certain points on the feet (and hands) correspond to parts of the body. Specific thumb, finger, and hand massage techniques are applied with varying degrees of pressure to the feet to promote well-being and healing. It is usual to concentrate on the feet rather than the hands. Foot massage has been practiced for thousands of years, but the term "zone therapy" was coined by Dr. William Fitzgerald in 1913. Eunice Ingham, who worked with Dr. Fitzgerald, developed his work. She carefully and precisely mapped the feet and all the areas of the body that corresponded when pressed. Ingham is recognized as the pioneer of modern reflexology, and she devoted over forty years of her life to the application and education of the system. After her death in 1974, Dwight Byers, her nephew, continued her life's work.

Although only apparently treating the feet, the whole body benefits and treatments should be profoundly soothing and calming. Practitioners who work with the chronically ill comment on its excellent ability to reduce tension and to promote deep relaxation, with the benefits extending well beyond the confines of the treatment. For patients struggling with chronic and serious conditions, weekly or fortnightly treatments are usual, but benefits are still felt with monthly treatments. To receive a treatment, the patient can rest, clothed except for the feet, with the shoulders and head supported and legs raised, while the therapist works on her feet.

Cancer Research UK conducted a study in 2007 where partners "gave reflexology to patients whose cancer had spread who had been taught by a qualified reflexologist. In the other group, the participants read to their partners for thirty minutes. The people who had reflexology had significantly less pain and anxiety." Although the study was carried out on only a small group of eighty-six people and further research is undoubtedly needed, it is now common to find reflexology offered by hospitals and hospices throughout the UK to patients suffering from chronic and severe pain. Reflexology is not recommended if you have blood clots in the leg veins, gout, foot ulcers, fungal conditions of the feet, epilepsy, or a very low platelet count that makes you bruise or bleed very easily.

My local community nurses referred me for such help in 2013 at a local hospital. The treatments proved enormously helpful when I was at such a low ebb. Again, you should seek out a fully qualified, experienced, and insured reflexologist, preferably one who has experience in dealing with the severely ill, as she will know that it is critical to only apply gentle pressure to the feet of people with chronic health conditions.

Reiki

> Energy cannot be created or destroyed; it can only
> be changed from one form to another.
> —Albert Einstein

Reiki is an energy healing system where the practitioner's hands are placed in various positions on, or slightly above, the client's body, and the client can be fully clothed during the treatment.

Although records demonstrate at least four other styles of hands-on healing systems in Japan at the start of the twentieth century, Mikao Usui, born in Japan in 1865, is credited with being the founder of the modern system of Reiki. He studied history, healing, Buddhism, and Taoism, and he was raised as a samurai from childhood, specifically in the martial art of aiki. Given an award by the Japanese government for doing honorable work to help others during his lifetime, he is often referred to as Usui Sensei, which means Master Usui in Japanese.

Chujiro Hayashi was born in 1880 in Tokyo and was a navy physician with a medical degree from the Imperial Japanese Naval Academy, graduating in 1902. He began to train with Dr. Usui in 1925 and was asked by Dr. Usui to continue his method and open a clinic in Tokyo. It was at this Tokyo clinic that Hawayo Takata started her Reiki training: Madam Takata was in fact native to Hawaii and on returning home brought Reiki to the United States and trained twenty-two Reiki masters in her system.

The thousands of Reiki practitioners throughout the West practicing Usui Ryoho (meaning Usui School) Reiki today can therefore trace their method directly back to Master Usui.

Reiki works primarily with energy centers in the body known as chakras, but also with meridians and the aura. Chakra is from the Sanskrit word *cakra*, meaning "wheel," and the concept of these energy centers throughout the body are present in Hindu, Buddhist, and Ayurvedic philosophical systems. They are also the basis for many forms of meditation practice and yoga: "These are whirling forces of subtle energy" (Finger 2018). A flow of energy is channeled down the arms of the practitioner into the client (never vice versa), and this activates and aligns the natural energy in the patient's body and cleanses and clears blockages in energy, thereby allowing it to flow freely. Studies of Reiki practitioners at work have "found that their hands emit a frequency between 7 Hz and 10 Hz" (Frazier 2018).

If the energy centers are considered small electrical sources within the body, then Reiki looks to recharge them as if they were small batteries. This in turn stimulates positive healing energy within the body. Reiki looks to "remove energetic blockages," "balance energy," and to "provide energetic support" (Frazier 2018).

During and after a treatment, patients often feel warm, deeply relaxed, and pleasantly sleepy. As lupus can feed on stress, such deep relaxation deprives it of this fuel.

A study of the implications of Reiki for forty university students with significant depression or anxiety and low depression and anxiety was carried out in 2011. After eight weeks, those who received treatment with Reiki had "progressive improvement in overall mood, while no change was seen in the control" (Bowden 2011). Clyde Norman Shealy, MD, PhD, a North American neurosurgeon, noted, "Reiki is one of the leading safe energy medicine approaches."

Reiki is not a diagnostic exercise. It works alongside orthodox treatment as a complementary therapy. Having previously experienced hands-on healing at the College of Psychic Studies in London, which has its own renowned and highly respected healing training program, I accepted Reiki when it was offered to me by a local hospital in 2013. In the National Health Service in the UK, Reiki is sometimes now offered as a complementary treatment to patients with chronic and severe medical conditions who are in crisis.

The IARP is the International Association of Reiki professionals, and it has been established for over twenty years, with thousands of members in over fifty countries. Further details on how to access its website and the websites of other leading training and regulatory bodies can be obtained in the resources section of this book.

The importance of massage, aromatherapy, reflexology, and Reiki is that they all complement mainstream medical treatment. In the right hands, they are gentle treatments that work to relax the body profoundly, imbue a sense of well-being, and provide layers of psychological and physical healing that are not provided by modern medicine.

The overarching principle that should apply to complementary physical treatments for lupus is that overly robust interventions from practitioners whose lack experience of working with long-term pain conditions can do more harm than good. Therapies that may work for generally healthy bodies can prove heavy-handed for lupus. Also, because lupus patients can look well when they are in fact fragile, it is easy for overenthusiastic practitioners to do too much.

They can instigate pain immediately or there is a danger of a delayed pain response. This is sometimes referred to as payback pain. Patients can also be overwhelmed by treatments and suffer fatigue and weakness hours, or a day or so, later. Given the dangers of triggered and payback pain with lupus sufferers, it is my experience that it is far better to try gentle treatments that work with the body rather than forcing, pummeling or manually adjusting it to any great degree.

During the course of my research, I have come across contraindications for mainstream chiropractic but not for the more gentle form, which is McTimoney chiropractic. In addition, osteopathy needs a highly experienced practitioner, and cranial osteopathy, which uses only the subtlest adjustments primarily to the head and sacrum, is preferred. You may come across a reluctance to treat long-term corticosteroid patients by chiropractors and osteopaths who may insist on evidence of a recent healthy DEXA bone density scan before they will proceed.

Given the fragile balance of the lupus system, it is also critical not to overlap or crowd therapies. Each should be given the appropriate space to work, and there needs to be room for the body to settle down between appointments. Piling two into one day, or on consecutive days, risks overwhelm. I would therefore advise a different complementary therapy every two weeks and no more than one per week; otherwise, there is a danger of overtreatment.

Appreciating that I have only referred to perhaps a few leading complementary therapies and that many others are available, further information on alternative therapies is in the resources section of the book. Whatever you try, I suggest that the following principles should apply to your chosen complementary therapy:

- The practitioners are experienced, registered and insured, and members of a leading regulatory body in their chosen field.
- They have specific experience in treating chronic pain and the severely ill.
- The approach is gentle and avoids heavy manipulation, kneading, or pummeling.
- It works complementary to modern medicine.
- Overlap and overtreatment is avoided.

Having made these caveats, it can be hugely beneficial if you source the right therapy and the right therapist, and an essential constituent of a successful, holistic approach to lupus. When in 2014, Lupus UK questioned 2,527 of its members, it noted in its summary of findings that almost a third, at 32 percent, "reported using alternative or complementary therapies, with acupuncture and massage being the most common."

I was referred to a physiotherapist in the autumn of 2016, and I explained to her exactly how careful I had to be, so to start with, she gave me some gentle stretching exercises that I was able to integrate gradually into my daily routine. These worked well at alleviating stiffness in my arms and legs, adding some extra flexibility, but I remained in pain.

I had also incorporated some hand stretching exercises kindly given to me by my neighbor Caroline, who is a physiotherapist, and they were proving to be beneficial for my stiff right hand in particular. The lupus in my central nervous system had partially damaged the nerves in my right hand, giving me numb patches across three fingers and half the palm. Luckily, there was no loss of functionality, just sensation. I also had to be careful of my thumb joints, which would swell regularly and be especially painful if I did too much. Overall, however, my hands were no longer the cramped claws that they had been. They could open out flat, and the fingers could straighten.

Reporting to my physio after a good Christmas, with fewer spikes in pain and nausea than the previous year, a new regime of more dynamic exercises was suggested. This new program included squats.

Unfortunately, within three days, this new set of exercises tipped my knees into an even higher level of pain. Now I was not only coping with generalized pain throughout my limbs and swelling on the knees, but also a new level of throbbing and burning. Nothing was able to make a difference to this extra pain, and it plagued me night and day. Despite the breath work and mindfulness, it interrupted my meditation practice and started to wear away at my overall progress.

Acupuncture

After three months, we started to consider acupuncture specifically to target the knees. My husband did some research for me and found a highly experienced practitioner locally, with a four-year degree in acupuncture and membership in the British Acupuncture Council. Jo's website also said that she had specific experience of autoimmune conditions and severe pain.

Acupuncture is arguably more than a complementary therapy; rather, it is part of a comprehensive Chinese health-care system that dates back at least 2,500 years. In China, it is quite usual for acupuncture hospitals to be sited close to Western medicine hospitals and for patients to visit both. The general theory is that energy flows throughout the body, and when disrupted or blocked, it leads to harmful symptoms and disease.

Through the insertion of very fine metal needles, painlessly, into certain points throughout the body, sometimes also with the addition of heat known as moxa, the correct flow can be stimulated, redirected, and restored. In the United States, acupuncture needles are regulated, just as are surgical equipment and hypodermic needles under good manufacturing and single-use sterility standards. I was familiar with acupuncture, had used it on several previous occasions, and knew it could be a useful and powerful technique. I just had concerns about tipping myself into further pain, nausea, or weakness, so it was with some trepidation that I went, desperate for any relief.

Two days after my first treatment with Jo, the pain in my knees reduced by 80 percent. Beyond thankful, I went for a series of fortnightly treatments, and the specific additional pain in my knees dissipated. Overall, apart from setbacks of spikes in pain and nausea when I still needed to inject to obtain relief, the pain in my legs also started to improve.

Then one morning, even before I opened my eyes, the awareness grew that something was different, very different. At first, I was perplexed. Half-asleep, I struggled to process what had changed. Then the realization hit: there was no pain. My body was stiff as I lay there, but otherwise nothing hurt. There was no stabbing, searing, aching, burning, throbbing, no underlying soreness even … just nothing. Tentatively, I lifted my head and then my shoulders off the pillows and shifted my legs toward the floor. Still nothing. Slipping into some clothes and gliding into the kitchen to make tea, I lifted the kettle with ease. While preparing breakfast, seemingly floating, the realization dawned that the incredible had happened: I was without pain for the first time in five years. Five years of continuous pain had finally stopped!

As the day progressed, the soreness returned, and not wanting to get carried away, I rested but went to bed that night excited at the prospect of waking once again pain-free. Not disappointed, the early morning of the second day took on a magical quality, with mindfulness simple as each task bathed in its own little golden glow of painlessness. I walked on air, feeling surreal; colors seemed brighter and the light sharper. I wrote NO PAIN! in capitals in my diary.

Four days later, I crashed. The soreness escalated rapidly, the nausea kicked in, and the searing pain renewed its grip. With the emergency routine enacted and an enforced return to the sofa, my confidence dived again. However, by the next morning, with the pain and weakness back under control, I took stock.

I reminded myself of all the physical ailments outrun, including severe liver damage, dysphagia, ascites, emaciation, discoid lesions, and hair loss. I reflected on the mental hurdles also jumped: despair, panic attacks, anxiety, depression, and obsessive thoughts. I reminded myself that winning against all of them had started with one single short breakthrough, which had then gathered momentum.

Now I knew this process was not linear and there was no clear map. Indeed, it would probably be erratic, frustrating, and even cruel, but I had been here before, survived, and made it through with my incredible support structure, taking one small step at a time. I'd compounded the positives and prevailed, despite repeated setbacks.

I knew that a precise route was not actually required to get there anyway. The door had been opened, and I had walked through it, however briefly, into a pain-free world. I believed completely that it had now been left ajar, and having done this once, I could do it again …

CONCLUSION

Suffering increases your inner strength.
—His Holiness the Dalai Lama

Part I illustrates why lupus is hard to diagnose and exposes the startling degree to which it is being belatedly diagnosed, misdiagnosed, and outright wrongly diagnosed. It expands on the view that there are people walking around today feeling unwell, who do not know that they have systemic lupus erythematosus.

It is for this reason that this book suggests that lupus may be a significant sleeper disease of modern times. It highlights the huge importance of continuing to raise awareness in order to improve the lives of those already diagnosed and to increase the wider understanding of what they face, but also to safeguard the health of those undiagnosed at this time.

To reduce the mystery and confusion surrounding lupus, part I clarifies the official route to diagnosis and conveys the history of the condition and its medical treatment, including the etymology of its strange name.

There is an increasing appreciation that the official eleven-point checklist of lupus symptoms still leaves room for false negatives and is not perhaps a gold standard in all cases. So just because a patient does not meet the criteria at a given time, this does not rule out systemic lupus erythematosus being present. Research into this continues.

As part of the process of giving a comprehensive understanding of what lupus entails, part I describes the key symptoms that are its hallmarks, aside from the official eleven-point checklist. This includes contributions from fellow lupus patients. It also lists the main medications used in the modern treatment of lupus and their leading physical and mental side effects.

There is currently no medication specifically designed for lupus or indeed for a whole set of related autoimmune conditions. This means that not only is there no cure at the present time, but with all the medications "borrowed" from other illnesses, prescriptions are often not an exact fit. They are therefore subject, as evidenced by my own journey as well as the testimony of fellow patients, to trial and adjustment.

As the renowned Johns Hopkins Lupus Center states on its website, "Lupus can be overwhelming and mysterious at times." The first four chapters are designed to provide clarity and to allay the bewilderment that I experienced and which I saw from my research is still being felt by others around the world.

Although fundamental, orthodox medicine is only part of a complete picture. In recognition of the profound psychological implications of this complex condition, the text advocates an approach that co-opts the mind. As Dr. Allen Lebovits, PhD, states, "The integration of psychological interventions with the treatment of chronic pain is essential."

The text also identifies the importance of having medical advisors you trust, who can give you confidence that you can and will make progress. As written: "You need to have faith in them and indeed they need to have faith in you." It examines the power of hope. Specifically, it counsels you to consider changes and to keep searching if you feel your needs are not being met.

The beginning of part II looks closely at the psychological implications of lupus, again including the experiences of other patients. It aims to verify and validate these emotions, some of which may chime with your own experience and allow you to say, "That is exactly how I feel!"

Referring to the latest research into how pain affects the brain, it explains why you are experiencing life like this, which may prove cathartic on its own. It shows that you have every right to feel stressed, depressed, and to think obsessively. It may allow you to stand back and say, "See, it's not me; it's my illness." This crucial awareness lays the basis for a way forward.

However, identifying that your reactions are justified still leaves you stuck with these negative emotions and behaviors, and it is acknowledged that this is a miserable and deeply troubling place to be. Ultimately, it is not doing your mind or your body any good.

In the search for resilience, part II goes on to suggest ways of breaking negative mental habits through proven and widely used cognitive behavioral methods. It offers tried-and-tested systems stemming from my training and experience as a counsellor and psychotherapist. These were the key building blocks to a change in my state of mind, despite my very severe lupus flare.

It proposes new practices for daily thinking and operating in order to create a momentous shift away from a negative, deeply unhappy state into a more constructive frame of mind. This methodology harnesses positive thinking to alter your internal dialogue radically.

It goes on to detail a system that promotes the pursuit of meaningful and absorbing projects to renew your sense of purpose. A method based on lists, daily tasks, and goal setting can renew your crushed feelings of achievement.

Developing this marked shift in perspective, this book aims to renovate further the understandable tendency for lupus to cause anxiety, worry, and panic, especially about our future, via breath work and the practice of mindfulness. The first stage of mindfulness looks to create a sense of calm in the moment, but its second phase seeks to erode ingrained negative response patterns, appreciate nature, and add beneficial rituals.

In addition, meditation is recommended to amplify the increasing sense of control and calm. Several forms of meditation and their history are discussed, but all those identified, if practiced regularly, will intensify the groundwork on positive thinking, new cognitive patterns, breath work, and mindfulness. Furthermore, it is recognized that positive visualizations will, despite the huge challenges of lupus, enhance an ability to live with relish and contentment. Ultimately, it cannot be overstated how important mental peace is to physical health and healing.

Overall, a holistic approach is recommended, wherein each part contributes something special to the healing process. It is rooted in widely respected methods, supported by the latest research, and has been practically applied and tested.

Nutrition is a fundamental building block of a holistic approach. Chapter 11 covers a balanced highly nutritious diet specifically tailored to the sensitivities and needs of lupus. The advice is broken down into the foods and beverages that can exacerbate lupus symptoms and the side effects of lupus medications, in addition to those that will ameliorate and improve both body and mind.

Then all these layers of medical, psychological, and nutritional understanding are enhanced by advice on body work, with a range of specially selected complementary solutions and therapies. The benefits of heat therapy, skilled and gentle massage, aromatherapy, reflexology, and Reiki are shown to provide levels of stress relief, relaxation, and healing that are not available elsewhere but which have been found to be essential for an effective approach to lupus. Finally, I reveal the role of acupuncture and how that specialized treatment capitalized on the solid platform that had been built gradually and carefully for five years, finally cracking my continuous cycle of pain.

In total, this book promotes a system providing clarity, resilience, and calm that has helped me to overcome many of the physical symptoms and psychological challenges posed by my severe lupus flare. Indeed, I am now able to face the prospect of an end to years of never-ending pain with joyful anticipation and a sense of robust equilibrium.

This narrative would be so much less were it not for the courage and honesty of others with lupus and comorbid autoimmune conditions who agreed to share their experiences in print, in the hope that it might help others facing this challenging condition.

I am also enormously grateful for the compassion and skill of my doctors and nurses along the way, often as part of our incredible National Health Service, for their immense help at low points and for the rescues that they have mounted on numerous occasions to deliver me from life-threatening situations, great pain, and distress.

In addition, I have recorded the knowledge and healing of my complementary therapists whose expertise and hands-on care has been applied with great diligence over weeks and months, patiently repairing me during my difficult journey.

Of incalculable value has been the unwavering support and immense kindness of my close family and friends. Pets also bring their own form of unconditional affection and healing, and I feel gratitude every day to have this structure around me, nestled in the heart of the English countryside.

I trust that this account contains something within its covers which is of use to you or a loved one. It has been written with the kindest intention and pure energy, and in this spirit, I truly hope that it helps you in your search for answers and a positive way forward.

REFERENCES

Chapter 2

"An overview of electromyography (EMG)".—Oxford Medicine
From *Atlas of Nerve Conduction Studies and Electromyography,* 2nd edition
A. A. Leis and M. P. Schenk
Available on: https://www.globaloup.com>product>atlas

"Systemic lupus erythematosus (SLE)".
C. M. Bartels, MD
November 14, 2017
Available on: http://www.medscape.com>articles

"How lupus affects the lungs".
Available on: https://www.hopkinslupus.org>lupus-info

"Cardiac involvement in systemic lupus erythematosus".
K. G. Moder et al.
Review Mayo Clinic Proceedings 1999
Available on: https://www.mayoclinicproceedings.org/article/S0025-6

"Oral lesions in lupus erythematosus: correlation with cutaneous lesions".
M. M. Nico et al.
June 23, 2008
Available on: https://www.researchgate.net>publication

"Photosensitivity and lupus".
National Resource Center on Lupus – Lupus Foundation of America
P. Werth, MD
March 2, 2017
Available on: https://www.resources.lupus.org>entry>light

"Lupus and sun exposure".

Written by the Healthline team and J. Bowman, medically reviewed by B. B. Spriggs, MD
July 21, 2016
Available on: https://www.healthline.com>health>lupus
Quote by kind permission of Ianrussell69
Lupus UK Forum
Available on: https://www.healthunlocked.com>lupus
"Biological false-positive tests for syphilis in the Jamaican population".
M. Smikle et al.
April 1990
Available on: https://www.ncbi.nlm.nih.gov.pubmed
"Venereal disease research laboratory test".
E. Hook in *Goldman's Cecil Medicine*, reported in ScienceDirect
Available on: https://www.sciencedirect.com>topics
"False-positive tests for HIV in a woman with lupus and renal failure".
R. Jindal et al.
Presented in the *New England Medical Journal*
April 29, 1993
Available on: https://www.nejm.org>doi>full>NEJ
"Seal: A lesson in lupus".
Available on: https://www.blackdoctor.org>pop-star-seal
"Subacute cutaneous lupus erythematosus: a decade's perspective".
R. D. Sontheimer
September 1989 and review 22 December 2017
Available on: https://www.ncbi.nlm.nih.gov>pubmed
"Who gets discoid lupus and can it turn into systemic lupus"?
Available on: https://www.kaleidoscopefightinglupus.org>whogetsdiscoid
lupus
"Patients with overlap autoimmune disease differ from those with "pure" disease".
M. Lockshin et al.
2015
Available on: https://www.lupus.bmj.com>content
The Lupus Foundation of America
Available on: https://www.lupus.org
"Sjögren's syndrome and lupus".

M. Lockshin
23 April 2012
Available on: https://www.hss.edu>conditionssjogrens
"Autoimmune disorder lupus may be triggered by body's bacteria".
J. Hamzelou
28 March 2018
Available on: https://www.newscientist.com>article
"Relationship between damage clustering and mortality in systemic lupus erythematosus in early and late stages of the disease".
J. M. Peigo-Reigosa
27 March 2016
Available on: https://www.ncbi.nlm.nih.gov>pubmed
"Study reveals shockingly high rates of incorrect lupus diagnosis".
By Lupus Foundation of America
4 November 2017
Available on: https://www.lupus.org/research-news/entry/study-reveals-high-rates-of-incorrect-lupus-diagnosis
"Summary of LUPUS UK member survey findings".
P. Howard
February 28, 2018
Available on: https://www.lupusuk.org.uk>member-survey
Chapter 3
"Lupus facts and statistics".—National Resource Center on Lupus
Lupus Foundation of America
2018
Available on: https://www.resources.lupus.org>entry>facts
"Ethnic disparities in patients with systemic lupus erythematosus".
A. G. Uribe, MD, and G. S. Alarçon, MD, Current Science Reports
2003
Available on https://www.link.springer.com
"The genetics of systemic lupus erythematosus".
R. H. Scofield
Available on: https://www.emedicine.medscape.com>article
"The enemy within: gut bacteria drive autoimmune disease".
March 8, 2018
M. Kriegel

Available on: https://www.news.yale.edu>2018/03/08>enemy
"The British Society for Rheumatology guidelines for the management of systemic lupus erythematosus in adults".
C. Gordon et al.
October 6, 2017
Available on: https://www.doi.org/10.1093/rheumatology/kex286
"Analysis of complete remission in systemic lupus erythematosus patients over a thirty-two-year period".
November 10, 2015
C. Medina-Quiñones et al. at the American College of Rheumatology
Available on: https://www.doi.org/10.1002/acr.22774
"Clinical approaches to management of background treatment in patients with SLE in clinical remission: results of an international survey".
March 2017
P. Ngamjanyaporn et al.
Quote with kind permission of AmyJ3
Lupus UK Forum
Available on: https://www.healthunlocked.com>lupus
The Chirurgia of Roger Frugard
L. D. Roseman, MD
Published by Xlibris
September 1, 2002
"Plaquenil: from malaria treatment to managing lupus".
C. Radis, DO
May 15, 2015
Available on: http://www.rheumatoidarthritis.net>treatment
Johns Hopkins Lupus Center
"A broader take on lupus".
May 1, 2013
Available on: http://www.hopkinslupus.org>lupus-treatment
"Living with lupus".
Lupus UK
Available on: https://www.lupusuk.org.uk
Quote by kind permission of Barnclown (Coco)
Lupus UK forum

Available on: https://www.healthunlocked.com>lupus
"Collagen diseases".
R. Kasukawa
2001
Available on: https://www.link.springer.com>chapter
"Mayo and the LE cell".
C. W. Nelson, Mayo Historical Unit
Available on: https://www.mayoclinicproceedings.org>hench
The London Lupus Centre
Available on: https://www.londonlupuscentre.co.uk
"The effect of hydroxychloroquine on the survival of patients with SLE: data from LUMINA, a multi-ethnic US cohort".
G. S. Alarcón et al.
March 27, 2007
Available on: https://ncbi.nlm.nih.gov>pubmed
"Eye screening for patients taking hydroxychloroquine (Plaquenil)".
The Royal College of Ophthalmologists
Available on: https://www.rcophth.ac.uk>2017/07>plaquenil
"Hydroxychloroquine retinopathy".
I. H. Yusuf et al.
10 March 2017
Available on: https://www.nature.com>eye>review
"Corticosteroids".
Johns Hopkins Lupus Center website
Available on: https://www.hopkinslupus.org>steroids
"Steroid-induced osteoporosis: how can it be avoided"?
P. M. Jehle
Nephrology Dialysis Transplantation, volume 18, issue 5, pages 861–864
May 1, 2003
Available on: https://academic.oup.com>ndt>article
"Cortosteroid-related central nervous system side effects".
M. Ciriaco et al.
December 4, 2013
Available on: https://www.ncbi.nlm.nih.gov-cortosteroid-relatedcentral nervoussystem
Chapter 4

"A Broader Take on Lupus".—Johns Hopkins Medicine
M. Hopkins, MD, Director Johns Hopkins Lupus Center
May 1, 2013
Available on: https://www.hopkinsmedicine.org>searchspring2013
Discovering the Body's Wisdom: A Comprehensive Guide to More Than Fifty Mind-Body Practices
M. Knaster
Published by Bantam New Age Books
1996
Quote with kind permission of Eliza
Personally interviewed May 2018
"Lupus fog: symptoms and causes".
The Mayo Clinic
Available on: https://www.mayoclinic.org>lupus>symptoms
"Lupus and the brain".
2011
D. B. Hellman, MD
Available on: https://www.lupusinternational.com>centralnervoussystem overview
"Esophageal disorders in lupus".
The National Resource Center for Lupus
Developed by the Lupus Foundation of America
Available on: https://www.resources.lupus.org.oesopheagealdisorders
"April's Topic of the Month—Coping with Hair Loss".
Lupus UK
P. Howard
April 27, 2016
Available on: https://www.lupusuk.org.uk>coping-with-hairloss
"Weather may truly affect arthritis pain".
S. Jegtvig
February 11, 2014
Available on: https://www.reuters.com>article>weather
"Fresh-faced (sunscreens)".
By I. Knight in the *Sunday Times* magazine
May 13, 2018
"A Guide to Pregnancy– Lupus UK".

Available on: https://www.resources.lupusuk.org.uk>2015/9

"Predisposition to cervical atypia in systemic lupus erythematosus: a clinical and cytopathological study".

H.H. Al Sherbeni et al.

Accepted January 26, 2015

Available on: https://www.hindawi.com/journals/ad/2015/751853/#B9

Chapter 5

"Prevalence of chronic pain in the UK: a systematic review and meta-analysis".

The British Medical Journal

A. Fayaz

June 20, 2016

Available on: https://www.bmjopen.bmj.com>content

"Functional magnetic resonance imaging".

S. A. Heuttal et al.

Published by Sinauer Associates 2009

Available on: https://www.journals.uchicago.edu>abs

"Chronic pain harms the brain".

D. Chialvo

February 5, 2008

Available on: https://www.northwesternedu>2008/02

"Chronic pain and depression are linked by brain gene changes".

A. Ananthaswamy

March 23, 2017

Available on: https://www.newscientist.com>article

"Undiagnosed mood disorders and sleep disturbances in primary care patients with chronic musculoskeletal pain".

A. Salazar

June 6, 2013

Available on: https://www.ncbi.nlm.nih.gov>pubmed

"The emotional and psychological impacts of chronic pain".

S. Moyle

February 3, 2016

Available on https://www.ausmed.com>articles>chronicpain

Quote with kind permission of Wendy39

Lupus UK Forum

Available on: https://www.healthunlocked.com>lupus
Invisible illness: "But you look so good."
Kaleidoscope Fighting Lupus/Living with Lupus
Available on: https://www.kaleidoscopefightinglupus.org>invisibleillness
"Self-conscious emotions in chronic musculoskeletal pain: a brief report".
J. Turner-Cobb et al.
January 2, 2015
Available on https://www.ncbi.nlm.nih.gov>articles
William Pitt the Younger: A Biography
By William Hague
1st edition, September 17, 2004
Published by Harper Press
"American Civilization"—*The Atlantic Magazine*
R. Waldo Emerson
April 1862 issue
Available on: https://www.theatlantic.com>1862>americancivilization
"Death's Homework".
P. J. O'Rourke—*The Guardian*, Opinion
October 7, 2008
Available on: https://www.theguardian.com>oct>healthandwell-being
"Undiagnosed mood disorders and sleep disturbances in primary care patients with chronic musculoskeletal pain".
A. Salazar et al.
Pain Medicine, volume 14, issue 9
September 1, 2013
Available on: https://www.doi.org/10.1111/pme.12165
"Prevalence of depression and anxiety in systemic lupus erythematosus: a systemic review and meta-analysis".
L. Zhang et al.
Published February 14, 2017
Available on: https://www.bmcpsychiatry.biomedicalcentral.com>prevalence
Chapter 6
Molly's Fund Fighting Lupus
Available on: https://www.kaleidoscopefightinglupus.org
Quote with kind permission of NadiaHJ

Lupus UK Forum
Available on: https://www.healthunlocked.com>lupus
Quote with kind permission of Leesy
Lupus UK Forum
Available on: https://www.healthunlocked.com>lupus
ICP Institute for Chronic Pain—"Ideas that are changing pain".
Founded by M. J. McAllister, PsyD
Available on: https://www.instituteforchronicpain.org
Quote with kind permission of Imom
Lupus UK Forum
Available on: https://www.healthunlocked.com>lupus
"Tips to get over your FOMO".
Dr. A. Gupta, PsyD
Available on: http://adaa.org>blog
Chapter 7
Cognitive Therapy and the Emotional Disorders
A. T. Beck
International Universities Press. Published 1976.
Cognitive Therapy of Depression
A. T. Beck et al.
The Guildford Press, New York. Published 1979.
Counselling for Stress Problems
S. Palmer and W. Dryden
Published by Sage, 1995.
"Change your thoughts, change your world".
J. R. Hawthorne
2014
Available on: https://www.jenniferhawthorne.com>articles.
Cognitive Therapy
D. Sanders and F. Wills
Sage Publications Ltd., 2nd edition. First published 2005.
Quote with kind permission of Horsewhisper
Lupus UK Forum
Available on: https://www.healthunlocked.com>lupus
Don't Believe Everything You Think: Living with Wisdom and Compassion
T. Chodron

January 8, 2013
Published by Snow, Lion, Boston & London
"Top 25 Positive Words, Phrases and Empathy Statements".
Published on February 14, 2018; last modified March 23, 2018
Available on: https://www.callcentrehelper.com
"Why rhyming phrases are more persuasive".
E. Inglis-Arkell
February 18, 2014
Available on: https://www.io9.gizmodo.com>whyrhyming-phrases
"Evolution of the human hand".
R. W. Young
Nov 22, 2002
Available on: https://www.ncbi.nlm.nih.gov>pubmed
"Did humans evolve opposable thumbs so we could punch each other"?
S. Fecht
October 21, 2015
Available on: https://www.popsci.com.did-our-oppos
The Complete Works of Swami Vivekananda
S. Vivekananda
2015
Published by Manonmani Publishers
Chapter 8
How to Get Things Done
D. Allen
Published by Piatkus, 1ˢᵗ edition 2001, revised 2015
"What's the point of being human? The best answer so far".
D. Chopra—The Blog
February 8, 2016; updated February 8, 2017
Available on: https://www.huffingtonpost.com>what's
"Study demonstrates that writing goals enhances goal achievement".
G. Matthews, PhD
Dominican University of California
Available on: https://www.dominican.edu>studydemonstrateswritinggoals
"How does distraction work in the management of pain"?
M. H. Johnson
Published April 2005

Available on: https://www.ncbi.nlm.nih.gov/pubmed

"Electronic gaming as a pain distraction".

E. Jameson MHSC et al.

Published in *Pain Research and Management*, January/February 2011

Available on: https://www.ncbi.nlm.nih.gov/pubmed

"Negative information weighs more heavily on the brain: the negative bias in evaluative categorizations".

T.A. Ito et al.

Journal of Personality and Social Psychology, vol. 75, October 1998

Available on: https://www.ncbi.nlm.nih.gov/pubmed

Laughter Therapy: How To Laugh About Everything In Your Life That Isn't Really Funny

A. Goodheart, PhD

Published by Less Stress Press, 1994

Sacred Space: Enhancing the Energy of Your Home and Office

D. Linn

2010

Published by Random House Books

"The big questions you face after a chronic illness diagnosis"

A. Dean

July 22, 2017

Available on: https://www.themighty.com

Chapter 9

The Art of Breathing

Dr. D. Penman

Harper Collins, 2016

The Relaxation Response

H. Benson, MD, with M. Z. Klipper

Revised edition 2001

Published by HarperCollins

Mindfulness for Beginners: Reclaiming The Present Moment And Your Life

J. Kabat-Zinn

Published by Sounds True 2012

Full Catastrophe Living: Revised Edition: How to cope with stress, pain and illness using mindfulness meditation

J. Kabat-Zinn

September 24, 2013
Published by Piatkus
The Mindfulness Bible: The Complete Guide to Living in the Moment
P. Collard
Published by Godsfield
"Mindfulness: a proposed operational definition".
S. R. Bishop et al.
University of Toronto
Clinical Psychology Science & Practice, Fall 2004
Available on: https://www.personal.kent.edu>bishop
Merriam-Webster Dictionary and Thesaurus
Available on: https://www.merriam-webster.com
Mindfulness for Beginners
G. Shaw
Kindle Edition
"Healing Wisdom: Healing Through Nature".
The Chopra Centre Radio S. McCabe and Dr. T. Bieske
T. Bieske, MD
April 6, 2011
Available on: https://www.blogtalkradio.com>2011/04/06
"The power of rituals in life, death, and business".
C. Nobel, Senior Editor of Harvard Business School Working Knowledge
Re: research by M. I. Norton and F. Gino
June 3, 2013
Available on: https://www.hbswk.hbs.edu>item>the-power
"Rituals enhance consumption".
K. Vohs et al.
August 17, 2018
Available on: https://www.harvard.edu/urn-3:HUL.InstRepos:10686852
The Buddha Pill: Can meditation actually change you?
Dr. M. Farias and C. Wikholm
May 2015
Published by Watkins
"Mind the hype: A critical evaluation and prescriptive agenda for research on mindfulness and meditation".
N. van Dam, M. van Vugt, and D. R. Vago

October 10, 2017
Available on https://www.doi.org/10.1177/174569617709589
"What is Mindfulness"? –The New Jersey Center for Mindful Awareness
Accessed on April 26, 2018
Available on: https://www.mindfulawarenessnj.com
Chapter 10
"Meditation programs for psychological stress and well-being: a systematic review and meta-analysis".
M. Goyal, MD, MPH
January 6, 2014
Available on: https://www.hub.jhu.edu>2014/01/08>meditation
"The neuroscience of mindfulness meditation".
S. McKay—The Chopra Center
Available on: https://www.chopra.com>articles>theneuroscienceof
"The neuroscience of mindfulness meditation".
Y. Y. Tang et al.
April 16, 2015
Available on: https://www.nature.com>nrn3916
Secrets of Meditation—A practical guide to inner peace and personal transformation
Davidj
Published by Hay House, 2012
"Progressive Relaxation: A physiological and clinical investigation of muscular states and their significance in psychology and medical practice".
E. Jacobsen, MD
Originally published 1929, Midway, reprint June 1, 1974
You Must Relax: A practical method of reducing the strains of modern living
E. Jacobsen, MD
Originally published 1934, 5th edition published in paperback March 1, 1978, by McGraw-Hill
"Deep progressive muscle relaxation technique for stress".
Essence of Stress Relief
Available on: https://www.essenceofstressrelief.com>progressivemuscle
"The power of visualization".

M. Neason
August 8, 2012
Sports Psychology Today
Available on: https://www.sportpsychologytoday.com>thepowerofvizualisation
Chapter 11
"Adult celiac disease followed by onset of lupus erythematosus"
H. J. Freeman
March 2008
Available on: https://www.ncbi.nlm.nih.gov>pubmed
"Is going gluten-free right for you"?
Dr. Christiane Northrup
Available on: https://www.drnorthrup.com>blog
"Nightshade vegetable sensitivity".
The Food Intolerance Institute of Australia
May 1, 2018
Available on https://www.foodintolerances.com/food-sensitivities/nightshades
"What to avoid with a nightshade allergy".
February 23, 2016
Available on: https://www.strengthandsunshine.com
"Critical evaluation of causality assessment of herb-drug interactions in patients".
British Journal of Clinical Pharmacology
January 24, 2018
C. Awortwe
Available on: https://www.bpspubs.onlinelibrary.wiley.com>herbs-drugs
"What's in ginkgo biloba and how does it work"?
ePainAssist
Reviewed by P. Kerkar, MD
Available on: https://www.epainassist.com>whatisginkgobiloba
"Advanced glycation end products".
P. Gkogkolou and M. Bohm
July 1, 2012
Available on: https://www.ncbi.nlm.nin.gov>pubmed
"The science of cooking oils: which really are the healthiest"?
C. Nierenberg
July 21, 2017

Available on: https://www.livescience.com>health
"Calcium and vitamin D for corto-steroid-induced osteoporosis".
J. Homik et al.
2000
Available on: https://www.ncbi.nlm.nin.gov>pubmed
"Steroid-induced osteoporosis: how can it be avoided"?
P. M. Jehle
2003
Available on: https://www.academic.oup.com>ndt>article
"What you need to know about anemia".
M. Rosove, MD
August 8, 2013
Available on: https://www.resources.lupus.org>entry>what
"Foods that fight inflammation".
Harvard Women's Health Watch
August 13, 2017
Available on https://www.health.harvard.edu>womens
"Top 15 anti-inflammatory foods".
Dr. Axe, Food is Medicine
Available on: https://www.draxe.com.autoimmunediseaseandimmunity
"What is hyperkalemia"?
National Kidney Foundation
Available on: https://www.kidney.org>hyperkalemia
"Randomised trial of analgesic effects of sucrose, glucose and pacifiers in terms of neonates".
R. Carbajal et al.
1999
Available on: https://www.ncbi.nlm.nin.gov/pubmed
"Effectiveness of sucrose analgesia in newborns undergoing painful medical procedures".
A. Taddio
2008
Available on: https://www.ncbi.nlm.nin.gov>pubmed
"The Fructose Overload".
Dr. Mercola's Natural Health Newsletter
Available on: https://www.mercola.com

"Sugar intake from sweet food and beverages, common mental disorder and depression: prospective findings from the Whitehall II study".
Dr. A. Knuppel et al.
July 27, 2017
Available on: https://www.researchgate.net>publication
"In vitro assessment of a honey bee pollen mix formulation".
E. Kuppeli Akkol et al.
March 2010
Available on: https://www.ncbi.nlm.nih.gov>pubmed
"Activities of different types of Thai honey on pathogenic bacteria causing skin diseases tyrosinase enzyme and generating free radicals".
K. Jantakee and Y. Tragoolpua
March 2010
Available on: https://ncbi.nlm.nin.gov>pubmed
"In vitro evaluation of antibacterial efficacy of pineapple extract (bromelain) on periodontal pathogens".
N. C. Praveen et al.
September 2014
Available on: https://ncbi.nlm.nin.gov>pubmed
"What is serotonin and what does it do"?
J. McIntosh
Feb 2, 2018
Available on: https://www.medicalnewstoday>serotoninandserotonin deficiency
"Dark chocolate consumption reduces stress and inflammation".
Loma Linda University Adventist Health Sciences Center
April 24, 2018
Available on: https://www.sciencedaily.com>2018/04
"Low-carb state of mind".—*Psychology Today*
Reviewed June 9, 2016
Available on: https://www.psychologytoday.com>low-carbstateofmind
"Is it possible to take too much vitamin C"?
K. Zeratsky, RD, LD
February 8, 2018
Available on: https://www.mayoclinic.org>vitaminc
"Magnesium: uses, side effects, interactions, dosage".

WebMD

Accessed 8 July 2018

Available on: https://www.webmd.com>vitamins>magnesium

"Anti-inflammatory properties of curcumin: a major constituent of curcuma longa: a review of preclinical and clinical research".

J. S. Jurenka

September 14, 2009

Available on: https://www.ncbi.nlm.nih.gov>pubmed

"Influence of piperine on the pharmacokinetics of curcumin and animals and human volunteers".

G. Shoba et al.

May 1998

Available on: https://www.ncbi.nlm.nih.gov>pubmed

Chapter 12

"How can a lack of touch lead to babies' failure to thrive"?

D. F. Bruce

March 27, 2015

Available on: https://www.sharecare.com/health/kids-teens-health/lack-of-touch-failure-to-thrive

"What is Qigong"?

The National Qigong Association

Available on: https://nqa.org>what-is-qigong

Aromatherapy An A–Z

P. Davis

Published by Random House Books

The Heart of Aromatherapy: An Easy-to-Use Guide for Essential Oils

A. Butje

2017

Published by Hay House

"Oxytocin hormone benefits and side effects".

R. Sahelian, MD

July 30, 2010

Available on https://www.scribd.com>document>oxytocin

"Perceived stress and cortisol levels predict speed of wound healing in healthy male adults".

M. Elbrecht et al.

June 16, 2003

Published in *Psychoneuroendocrinology* (2004) 798–809

Available on: https://www.ncbi.nlm.nih.gov>pubmed

Reflexology quote by kind permission of R. Bickerton

September 6, 2018

Available on: https://www.handsonfeet.com

"Reflexology/Cancer in General/Cancer Research UK".

Study 2007

Available on: https://www.cancerresearchuk.org>reflexology

"Chakras 101—what exactly are these whirling forces of energy"?

Y. A. Finger

January 18, 2018

Available on: https://www.yogajournal.com>videos

Reiki Healing for Beginners: The Practical Guide with Remedies for 100+ Ailments

K. Frazier

2018

Published by Althea Press

"A randomized controlled single-blind trial of the efficacy of Reiki at benefitting mood and well-being".

March 27, 2011

D. Bowden et al.

Available on: https://www.ncbi.nlm.nih.gov>articles

"Summary of Lupus UK Membership Findings".

P. Howard

February 28, 2018

Available on: https://www.lupusuk.org>member-survey

RECOMMENDED READING

Sacred Space: Enhancing the Energy of your Home and Office
By Denise Linn
Published by Random House Books 2010

Power Thoughts: 365 Daily Affirmations
By Louise L. Hay
Published by Hay House 2005

Getting Things Done: The Art of Stress-Free Productivity
By David Allen
Published by Piatkus 2nd edition 2015

The Art of Breathing
By Danny Penman
Published by Harper Collins 2016

The Mindfulness Bible
By Patrizia Collard
Published by Godsfield

Buddhism: A Practical Guide to Integrating and Practicing Buddhism in Everyday Life
By Will Huyn
Published by Will Huyn 2015

Secrets of Meditation: A Practical Guide to Inner Peace and Personal Transformation
By Davidji
Published by Hay House 2012

Transcendental Meditation: The Essential Teachings of the Maharishi Mahesh Yogi
By Jack Forem
Published by Hay House Revised Edition 2012

Happy for No Reason: 7 Steps to Being Happy from the Inside Out
By Marci Shimoff
Published by Free Press, a Division of Simon & Shuster 2008
Discovering the Body's Wisdom: A Comprehensive Guide to More Than 50 Mind-Body Practices
By Mirka Knaster
Published by Bantam Books 1996
The Heart of Aromatherapy: An Easy-to-Use Guide for Essential Oils
By Andrea Butje
Published by Hay House 2017
Reiki Healing for Beginners: The Practical Guide with Remedies for 100+ Ailments
By Karen Frazier
Published by Althea Press 2018
Goddesses Never Age: The Secret Prescription for Radiance, Vitality, and Well-Being
By Dr. Christiane Northrup
Published by Hay House 2015

USEFUL WEBSITES

The Lupus Foundation of America
Available on: https://www.lupus.org
John's Hopkins Lupus Center
Available on: https://www.hopkinslupus.org
St. Thomas' Lupus Trust
Available on: https://www.lupus.org.uk
The London Lupus Centre
For Hughes syndrome
Available on: https://www.thelondonlupuscentre.co.uk
LUPUS UK HealthUnlocked
Support Forum for Lupus
Available on: https://www.healthunlocked.com>lupusuk
The Complementary Therapists Association
Available on: https://www.ctha.com
The General Osteopathic Council
Available on: https://www.osteopathy.org.uk
The British Acupuncture Council
Available on: https://acupuncture.org.uk
The Aromahead Institute
Available on: https://www.aromahead.com
The Aromatherapy Council
Available on: https://www.aromatherapycouncil.org.uk
The International Association for Reiki Professionals
Available on: https://www.iarp.org
The Reiki Council
Available on: https://www.reikicouncil.org.uk
The Reiki Guild

Available on: https://www.reikiguild.co.uk
Louise Hay
Available on: https://www.louisehay.com
The Chopra Center
Available on: https://chopra.com
Davidji
Available on: https://davidji.com
Davidji Guided Meditations
Available on: https://www.davidji.com>meditation>free-guided-meditations
Paraliminal Learning Strategies Audio Programs
Available on: https://www.learningstrategies.com

A

ketchup 127
ketogenic 139
kidneys 7, 10, 11, 27, 32, 35, 36, 51, 54,
      129, 131, 133, 134, 147, 179

L

lactobacillus 131
lactose 131
lamb 130, 133, 134, 140
lavender 146, 150, 151
laxatives 141, 143
L-canavanine 129
leflunomide 49
lemon 150
lentils 131, 132, 139
leopard 13
lesions 8, 12, 13, 25, 49, 159, 165
lethargy 62
lettuce 133
leukemia 22
lifting 72, 99, 100, 110
lighting 9, 67, 72
lime 150
linalool 151
linens 45
lips 15, 16, 53, 64, 142
low-carbohydrate 139
low-potassium 134
low-sodium 127, 134
lucidity 42
lumbar 130
lungs 7, 8, 22, 27, 32, 103, 104, 107, 133,
      151, 165
lycopene 133
lymphatic 25

M

mackerel 133
magnesium 137, 141, 143, 146, 147,
      180, 181
malar 7, 12, 13, 25, 64

malaria 26, 27, 32, 45, 168
mangos 133
manicures 35
mantra 86, 117
masseuse 148
McTimoney 156
Medina-Quiñones 24, 168
melatonin 139
melons 133
meningitis 17
Menstrual 72
mepacrine 36
meridians 155
methotrexate 35, 49
methylprednisolone 33
migraines 9, 10, 31
milk 34, 47, 131
mini-flares 73, 83, 88, 115, 148
miscarriages 31, 51, 150
misdiagnosed 17, 161
misdiagnosis ix, 16
mofetil 36, 54, 55
molar 51
molasses 132
mononucleosis 23
morphine 36, 41, 42, 43, 45, 148
mosquitos 27
moxa 158
mozzarella 48
MRI 2, 10, 60
MS 98
muscular dystrophy 22
musculoskeletal 62, 171, 172
myalgic 14
mycophenolate 36, 54, 55, 69

N

nails 35, 142
Naprosyn 32
naproxen 32
narcoleptic 36, 45, 128

pineal 148
piperine 181
pituitary 147
plaques 8
platelet 10, 154
pleiotropic 144
pleura 8
pneumonitis 8
pollen 137, 180
potassium 133, 134, 137, 141
potato 126, 127, 133, 139
poultry 130, 134, 135, 140
pox 35
prednisolone 15, 33, 34, 54, 68
preeclampsia 31
pregnancy x, 31, 51, 53, 150, 151, 170
premenstrual 52
preservative 16, 129
probiotic 143, 144
propolis 137
protuberant 14
prune 132
psoriasis 14, 146
Psychoneuroendocrinology 182
psychosomatic 17
pulmonary 8
pumpkin 132

Q

Qigong 148, 181
quinacrine 32
quinine 26, 27
quinoa 132

R

ranitidine 34, 54
raspberries 133
Raynaud's 14, 15, 22, 24, 35, 147
rays 9, 10, 34, 50, 70, 149
RDA 142, 143
reagin 30

redness 15
reflux 48
Renal 7, 10, 166
respiratory 137, 151
retinal 33
retinopathy 33, 169
reuptake 128
rheumatologist 24, 36, 51, 70, 77
Rheumatology 7, 23, 24, 168
rice 132, 138, 139
rigid 2, 40, 41, 118, 148
risottos 135
rituximab 36
Rogerius 25
Rose 152
Rosemary 152
rye 126, 139
Ryoho 155

S

sacrum 156
saliva 15, 16, 51, 141
salmon 130, 131, 133, 139
salsas 127
salt 127, 128, 141, 143, 144, 146, 147
samurai 154
Sanskrit 155
sardines 131, 132, 133
scalp 49
scars 12, 13, 143
sclerosis 14, 22, 149
Seafood 130
Seal x, 12, 166
seaweed 139
sedation 60
sedimentation 10
seizures 12, 46
selenium 137
self-awareness 100
self-blaming 81
self-criticize 85

W

X

Y

Z

ACKNOWLEDGMENTS

I am hugely thankful to the many people who were prepared to share their deeply personal experiences with me to benefit this book, and to those who gave years of knowledge, insight, and expertise freely in order to increase the understanding of lupus.

In particular, I would like to thank those who gave me permission to quote their words directly (in the order that they appear), namely Ian, Amy, Coco, Eliza, Wendy, Nadia, Leesy, Imom, Horsewhisper, and Rosanna Bickerton.

I feel deeply grateful for the wonderful help, support, and kindness I have received from family, friends, and professionals along my lupus journey, but in particular, I would like to thank the following:

Dr. Raffi Assadourian
Lisa and Mark Bartlett
Julie Bond
Ashley Edwards
Nicola Eldridge
Sheila Freakins
Dr. Phillip Harrison
Juliet and Andrew Henderson
Dr. Wendy Holden
Jo Lewis
Dale McDougall
Angela McGown

Mary Nardulli
Mark Neve
Dr. Claudia Shand
Patricia Stephen
Michael and Tina Tomlin
Hayley Wells

Karen has an MA (Hons) in English Literature from the University of St Andrews in Scotland. Her first career was in finance, and she worked in the City of London as a stockbroker and asset manager. Her roles included head of research, divisional director of asset management, and chief investment officer. She retrained as a counsellor and psychotherapist, qualifying with distinction, and is an accredited member of the National Counselling Society.

She worked for two leading mental health charities, for a mental health development service, and with young people with complex disabilities, before falling seriously ill in 2012 with a severe lupus flare. She writes, counsels, and speaks about chronic pain and illness. She lives in the heart of the English countryside with her husband and their dogs.

9 781982 220495